CORE
REVIEW
FOR
CRITICAL
CARE
NURSING

Editors

SUSAN WILLIAMS, R.N., M.S.N., CCRN

Assistant Professor, Critical Care Nursing,
Department of Graduate Studies and Research,
College of Nursing, Northwestern State University of Louisiana,
Shreveport, Louisiana

JoANN GRIF ALSPACH, R.N., M.S.N., CCRN

Nursing Education Consultant, Critical Care,
Annapolis, Maryland

W. B. SAUNDERS COMPANY

Philadelphia, London, Toronto, Mexico City, Rio de Janeiro, Sydney, Tokyo, Hong Kong

W. B. SAUNDERS COMPANY
Harcourt Brace Jovanovich, Inc.

The Curtis Center
Independence Square West
Philadelphia, PA 19106

Library of Congress Cataloging in Publication Data

Main entry under title:

Core review for critical care nursing.

1. Intensive care nursing—Addresses, essays, lectures.
   I. Williams, Susan, 1942–   II. Alspach, JoAnn.
   [DNLM: 1. Critical Care—nurses' instruction. WY 154 C797]

RT120.I5C67 1985   610.73'61   84–29836

ISBN 0–7216–1142–7

Core Review for Critical Care Nursing   ISBN   0–7216–1142–7

Last digit is the print number: 9   8   7   6   5

CONTRIBUTORS

CHAROLD L. BAER, R.N., Ph.D.

Professor, Department of Adult Health and Illness, School of Nursing, Oregon Health Sciences University, Portland, Oregon.

HELEN BAIRD, R.N., M.S.N.

Psychiatric Clinical Nurse Specialist, Clinical Instructor to Department of Psychiatry, LSU Medical School, Northwestern State University, Department of Nursing, Shreveport, Louisiana.

DIANE K. DRESSLER, R.N., M.S.N., CCRN

Clinical Nurse Specialist, Midwest Heart Surgery Institute, Milwaukee, Wisconsin.

MAURENE A. HARVEY, R.N., M.P.H., CCRN

Educational Consultant, Consultants in Critical Care, Inc., Glendale, California.

NANCY M. HOLLOWAY, R.N., M.S.N., CCRN, C.E.N.

Nancy Holloway and Associates, Inc., Oakland California.

TERESA THOMA KEVIL, R.N., M.N.Sc., C.N.S.

Assistant Professor of Nursing, Northwestern State University, College of Nursing, Shreveport, Louisiana.

SUSAN ARMSTRONG SCREWS, R.N., M.N.Sc., C.N.S.

Assistant Administrator for Nursing, Louisiana State University Medical Center, Shreveport, Louisiana.

PREFACE

The CORE REVIEW FOR CRITICAL CARE NURSING is designed to be a self-assessment of knowledge important to the practice of modern critical care nursing. The text has been developed to provide a useful study guide in conjunction with the current (third) edition of CORE CURRICULUM FOR CRITICAL CARE NURSING. When used in this manner, the companion volumes provide not only an outline of currently accepted nursing theory and practice but also application of this information. The contributors have made special efforts to ensure that the questions are accurate and reflect the most important aspects of the CORE CURRICULUM.

The format for this study guide is multiple-choice. We believe that this format offers the most versatile means for the evaluation of knowledge and that it also has the advantage of letting the reader become familiar with standardized test-taking. Four options are presented with each item; the reader is instructed to choose the best one. Immediate feedback is provided and the book's value as a self-testing tool is enhanced by having the correct answer identified two pages after the question (for example, questions on page 31 are answered on page 33; questions on page 32 are answered on page 34). The reader is also given the rationale for the correct choice as well as the reason that the incorrect answers are not appropriate, when warranted.

There are a total of 750 items in the text, with each chapter corresponding to the companion chapter of the third edition of CORE CURRICULUM FOR CRITICAL CARE NURSING. Because they represent the major pathologic disorders seen in the critically ill patient, the pulmonary and cardiovascular systems chapters have the most items alloted to them, 150 each. The remaining chapters (neurologic, renal, gastrointestinal, hematologic, endocrine, and psycho-social implications) have 75 items each. Within each chapter, the distribution of items is consistent with the distribution of content in the CORE CURRICULUM FOR CRITICAL CARE NURSING, third edition. The questions were written with an emphasis on application of knowledge, integration of facts, and under-standing of basic concepts.

Although CORE CURRICULUM FOR CRITICAL CARE NURSING, third edition, was the primary source for the text, other references were used by the contributors in preparation of the items. They are listed at the end of each chapter and serve as additional instructional material for the reader.

CORE REVIEW FOR CRITICAL CARE NURSING was written for practicing critical care nurses, nursing educators, and students. It may also be useful as one of a number of references to review in preparation for the CCRN examination. We welcome your comments and suggestions.

SUSAN M. WILLIAMS

JOANN GRIF ALSPACH

ACKNOWLEDGMENTS

Many individuals have contributed to the development of the CORE RE-VIEW FOR CRITICAL CARE NURSING. This self-study book, a companion volume to ACCN'S CORE CURRICULUM FOR CRITICAL CARE NURS-ING, had been discussed for some time by the AACN Board of Directors and Publications Committee. These groups have provided the support and guidance necessary to bring the project into realization. Individual contributors worked tirelessly to develop and refine the test items, rationales, and references for each chapter. Several worked under very tight schedules as the project neared comple-tion, and for their efforts we are deeply grateful.

To ensure both accuracy and relevance of content, each chapter was reviewed by nurse and physician experts, whose names appear on the next page. They deserve our special thanks for giving freely of their time. We would also like to thank the secretaries at Louisiana State University Medical Center and North-western State University College of Nursing in Shreveport.

Finally, we thank our husbands, Darryl and Rodger, and our children, Carol, Peter, Sarah, and Jenny, for their continued support and patience during the past year.

CHAPTER REVIEWERS

1. THE PULMONARY SYSTEM

Mary Ellen Wewers, R.N., M.N.Sc., Pulmonary Clinical Nurse Specialist, Doctoral Candidate, University of Maryland School of Nursing, University Park, Maryland.

Gary T. Kinasewitz, M.D., Associate Professor of Medicine, Physiology, and Biophysics, Departments of Medicine, Physiology, and Biophysics, Louisiana State University School of Medicine, Shreveport, Louisiana.

2. THE CARDIOVASCULAR SYSTEM

Sharon Walters Walker, R.N., M.S.N., C.N.S., Associate Director of Critical Care, Bossier Medical Center, Bossier City, Louisiana.

William J. Bugni, M.D., F.A.C.C., Assistant Professor of Medicine, University of South Florida College of Medicine; Director, Cardiac Catheterization Lab, James A. Haley Veterans Administration Medical Center, Tampa, Florida.

3. THE NEUROLOGIC SYSTEM

Ellen B. Rudy, R.N., Ph.D., Associate Professor, School of Nursing, and Program Director, Nursing of the Adult Graduate Program, Kent State University, Kent, Ohio.

Jacquelin S. Neatherlin, R.N., M.S.N. C.N.R.N., Head Nurse, Neuro-Med-Surg Floor, Harris Hospital Methodist, Fort Worth, Texas.

Edward Benzel, M.D., Chief, Division of Neurosurgery, and Assistant Professor, Louisiana State University School of Medicine, Shreveport, Louisiana.

4. THE RENAL SYSTEM

Larry E. Lancaster, R.N., Ed.D., Associate Professor and Academic Director, Graduate Medical-Surgical Clinical Major, School of Nursing, Vanderbilt University, Nashville, Tennessee.

June L. Stark, R.N., B.S.N., CCRN, Critical Care Instructor and Renal Nurse Consultant, New England Medical Center, Boston, Massachusetts.

George A. DeVault Jr., M.D., Assistant Professor, Department of Medicine, Section of Nephrology and Hypertension, Louisiana State University Medical Center, Shreveport, Louisiana.

5. THE ENDOCRINE SYSTEM

Patricia Caudle, R.N.P., M.N.Sc., C.F.N.P., Assistant Professor, Department of Graduate Studies and Research in Nursing, Family Nurse Clinician Track, Northwestern State University, College of Nursing, Shreveport, Louisiana.

Joseph Loewenstein, M.D., Professor of Medicine, Section of Endocrinology, Louisiana State University School of Medicine, Shreveport, Louisiana.

6. THE HEMATOLOGIC SYSTEM

Ann Blattner, R.N., M.S.N., Nurse Coordinator–Radiation Oncology, Mount Sinai Medical Center, Milwaukee, Wisconsin.

Robert F. Taylor, M.D., Medical Consultants, Ltd., Private Practice in Hematology and Medical Oncology, Milwaukee, Wisconsin.

7. THE GASTROINTESTINAL SYSTEM

Susan VanDeVelde-Coke, R.N., M.A., M.B.A., Director of Nursing, Health Science Center General Hospital, Winnipeg, Manitoba, Canada.

Catherine V. Netchvolodoff, M.D., Gastroenterologist, Veterans Administration Medical Center; Assistant Professor, Department of Medicine, Louisiana State University School of Medicine, Shreveport, Louisiana.

8. PSYCHOLOGICAL IMPLICATIONS

Carol G. Scott, R.N., M.S.N., Instructor, Critical Care Nursing, Lynchburg General and Marshall Lodge Hospitals School of Nursing, Lynchburg, Virginia.

Robert McConnell Young, M.D., Psychiatrist; Acting Director, Mental Health and Substance Abuse Clinic, Minden, Louisiana.

CONTENTS

HOW TO USE THIS BOOK

HOW TO USE THIS BOOK

To better help you to use this book for self-testing, answers are not given on the page on which the questions are asked. Instead, the answers to questions on an odd-numbered page appear on the next odd-numbered page, and questions on an even-numbered page are answered on the next even-numbered page.

Questions are always given in the left-hand column of the page. Answers are always in the right-hand column. A box at the top of the "Answers" column refers you to the page number of the relevant questions.

1□ THE PULMONARY SYSTEM

TERESA THOMA KEVIL
SUSAN ARMSTRONG SCREWS

1. Oxygen and carbon dioxide are exchanged between the

   A. Alveoli and arterioles.
   B. Bronchioles and vena cavae.
   C. Alveoli and pulmonary capillaries.
   D. Bronchioles and abdominal aorta.

2. *Respiratory quotient* refers to internal or cellular respiration and reflects the ratio of

   A. The fraction of inspired oxygen (FI_{O_2}) to the serum glucose level.
   B. The FI_{O_2} to oxygen consumed.
   C. Ingested carbohydrates to ingested fats.
   D. Carbon dioxide produced to oxygen consumed.

3. External respiration, or the exchange of O_2 and CO_2 at the alveolar-capillary level, is measured by

   A. Determining the ratio of CO_2 produced to O_2 taken up per minute.
   B. Subtracting the Pa_{O_2} from the FIO_2.
   C. Subtracting the Pa_{CO_2} from the Pa_{O_2}.
   D. Determining the ratio of O_2 consumed to CO_2 produced.

4. The three primary interactive systems that allow for proper functioning of the respiratory circuit are the respiratory system, cardiovascular system, and

   A. Renal system.
   B. Gastrointestinal system.
   C. Integumentary system.
   D. Neuromuscular system.

5. The area of the respiratory tree where gas flows, but is not exchanged, is called

   A. Atelectasis.
   B. Anatomic dead space.
   C. Interstitial infarction.
   D. Bronchiectasis.

6. Endotracheal intubation or tracheostomy negates the upper protective function of

   A. Cooling the air.
   B. Filtering the air.
   C. Drying the air.
   D. Volumetric control of the air.

7. When a person swallows, the larynx responds by

   A. Closing the glottis.
   B. Opening the epiglottis.
   C. Forcing air to vibrate the vocal cords.
   D. Stimulating sensory fibers to signal the superior laryngeal nerve.

8. The part of a child's anatomy that eliminates the need for a cuffed endotracheal tube is the

   A. Thyroid cartilage.
   B. Arytenoid cartilage.
   C. Alar cartilage.
   D. Cricoid cartilage.

9. The finding of normal breath sounds on the right chest and diminished, distant breath sounds on the left chest of a newly intubated patient is probably due to

   A. A left pneumothorax.
   B. A right hemothorax.
   C. Intubation of the right mainstem bronchus.
   D. A malfunctioning mechanical ventilator.

10. The site in the bronchial tree most sensitive to CO_2 levels is the

    A. Terminal bronchioles.
    B. Carina.
    C. Right mainstem bronchus.
    D. Left mainstem bronchus.

11. The alveolar cells that are associated with the synthesis of surfactant are the

    A. Type I cells.
    B. Type II cells.
    C. Type III cells.
    D. Alveolar macrophages.

12. Pulmonary surfactant

 A. Insures an unvarying surface tension.
 B. Reduces lung compliance.
 C. Varies surface tension with changes in alveolar volume.
 D. Enhances atelectasis during expiration.

13. The lung is in contact with approximately 60 to 140 ml of pulmonary capillary blood at any one time because the alveolocapillary membrane lines alveolar ducts, alveolar sacs, alveoli, and

 A. The trachea.
 B. The carina.
 C. Respiratory bronchioles.
 D. Segmental bronchi.

14. The minute ventilation ($\dot{V}_E$), which is the amount of air breathed in 1 minute, can be measured by

 A. Multiplying the exhaled tidal volume (V_T) by the respiratory rate (f).
 B. Subtracting the expiratory reserve volume (ERV) from the tidal volume (V_T).
 C. Dividing the tidal volume (V_T) by the physiologic dead space ($\dot{V}_D$).
 D. Adding the inspiratory reserve volume (IRV) to the expiratory reserve volume (ERV).

15. A 120-lb female is ventilated 10 times per minute with a tidal volume of 600 ml. Her minute ventilation is

 A. 5.5 L.
 B. 6 L.
 C. 7 L.
 D. 8.25 L.

16. A 190-lb male is admitted to the ICU, intubated, and placed on a mechanical ventilator with an $F_{I_{O_2}}$ of 0.4, tidal volume of 800, and rate of 12. What is his minute alveolar ventilation?

 A. 660 ml.
 B. 2928 ml.
 C. 7320 ml.
 D. 9600 ml.

Answers to Questions from page 1

1. (**C**) The exchange of oxygen and carbon dioxide to and from the atmosphere involves the alveoli. The exchange between the lungs and systemic circulation occurs between the alveoli and pulmonary capillaries. Alveoli are also lined with an alveolar-capillary membrane, which allows exchange of gas between alveoli and pulmonary capillaries.

2. (**D**) The respiratory quotient varies, depending on the composition of ingested food. It is estimated by the ratio of CO_2 produced to O_2 consumed ($\dot{V}_{CO_2}/\dot{V}_{O_2}$) and normally is about 0.8.

3. (**A**) External respiration is measured by the respiratory exchange ratio, which is the ratio of CO_2 produced to O_2 taken up per minute. In a homeostatic state, the amount of CO_2 produced by the tissues will equal the amount of CO_2 excreted by the lungs. Under the same conditions, the amount of O_2 consumed is balanced by the amount of O_2 taken up per minute. Therefore, this ratio is normally 0.8.

4. (**D**) The neuromuscular system is integral for proper functioning of the respiratory circuit. The brain responds to changes in systemic oxyen requirements (e.g., due to altered activity levels or environmental changes) by sending impulses via the neuromuscular system that initiate compensatory maneuvers.

5. (**B**) Anatomic dead space includes the entire area from nose to respiratory bronchioles where gas flows but is not exchanged. It usually amounts to about 2 ml/kg body weight. *Atelectasis* refers to collapse of alveoli. *Bronchiectasis* refers to an inflammatory or degenerative condition of bronchi or bronchioles.

17. The relationship between the partial pressure of arterial CO_2 (Pa_{CO_2}) and alveolar ventilation ($\dot{V}_A$) is

    A. Insignificant, because these two parameters are unrelated.
    B. Inversely proportional (i.e., $\uparrow \dot{V}_A = \downarrow Pa_{CO_2}$).
    C. Directly proportional (i.e., $\uparrow \dot{V}_A = \uparrow Pa_{CO_2}$).
    D. One of equality at all times (i.e., $\dot{V}_A$ always equals Pa_{CO_2}).

18. The antigen stimulation of humoral and cell-mediated immune systems that adds immunoglobins to the surface fluid of alveoli will activate

    A. Alveolar macrophages.
    B. Cilia motion.
    C. Gas exchange.
    D. Fluid production.

19. The primary muscle(s) of resting or quiet respiration is (are) the

    A. Intercostals.
    B. Diaphragm.
    C. Pectoralis major.
    D. Sternocleidomastoid.

20. A major difference between expiration and inspiration is that expiration is

    A. An active act.
    B. Usually forced.
    C. Energy consuming.
    D. A passive act.

21. The action of muscles during the respiratory cycle facilitates the movement of air into and out of the lungs by

    A. Stimulating the heart to better perfuse the lungs.
    B. Altering intrathoracic pressures in relationship to atmospheric pressure.
    C. Increasing pulmonary oxygen consumption.
    D. Sending impulses to the hypothalamus.

22. When a lung is stiff and resists distention, there is low

    A. Airway resistance.
    B. Compliance.
    C. Transthoracic resistance.
    D. Hypoxemia.

Answers to Questions from page 2

6. **(B)** The respiratory protective functions of the upper airway are to filter, warm, and humidify the air. These protective functions are negated when these passages are bypassed, as with an endotracheal or tracheostomy tube.

7. **(A)** When a person swallows, the epiglottis snaps closed, thereby closing off the glottis and helping to prevent aspiration. Phonation or speech results from vibration of the vocal cords by expired air. The superior laryngeal nerve is one of two branches of the vagus nerve that innervate the larynx. Stimulation of the laryngeal nerve results in the cough reflex.

8. **(D)** The cricoid cartilage is a complete ring and the narrowest part of a child's airway. Thus, a cuffed endotracheal tube is unnecessary for a child.

9. **(C)** The right mainstem bronchus is shorter, wider, and more in line with the trachea than the left mainstem bronchus. As a result, it is not uncommon for the endotracheal tube to be advanced beyond the carina, resulting in right mainstem bronchus intubation. This condition can be confirmed by radiographic and auscultatory assessment; it is remedied by repositioning the tube above the carina.

10. **(A)** Terminal bronchioles respond to increased CO_2 levels by dilating; they respond to decreased CO_2 levels by constricting.

11. **(B)** Type II cells are metabolically active, secretory cells associated with the synthesis of surfactant. Type I cells are involved in gas exchange and in inhibition of fluid transudation into the alveoli. Alveolar macrophages are phagocytic cells.

23. A patient is admitted to the hospital with unusually low rate and depth of respiration. This condition may be due to a dysfunction in the

    A. Cerebrum.
    B. Cerebellum.
    C. Medulla.
    D. Thalamus.

24. It is postulated that a prolonged, deep inspiration is initiated by the

    A. Apneustic center.
    B. Pneumotaxic center.
    C. Hypophysis.
    D. Cerebral cortex.

25. A 70-kg patient admitted with a head injury has a tidal volume of 500 ml and a respiratory rate of 10 per minute. What is his minute ventilation?

    A. 50 ml.
    B. 5000 ml.
    C. 1000 ml.
    D. 35,000 ml.

26. The same patient as in question 25 has a Pa_{CO_2} of 50 mm Hg. What can be concluded about his alveolar ventilation?

    A. Alveolar ventilation is decreased.
    B. Alveolar ventilation is increased.
    C. Alveolar ventilation is normal.
    D. Alveolar ventilation is unrelated to Pa_{CO_2}.

27. If a patient suffers an inhalation injury that results in alveolocapillary membrane damage, which of the following is most likely?

    A. A low Pa_{O_2}.
    B. A high Pa_{CO_2}.
    C. A high sedimentation rate.
    D. A low white blood cell count.

Answers to Questions from page 3

12. **(C)** Surfactant allows for variation in surface tension related to alveolar volume, thus reducing the possibility of atelectasis by keeping alveoli open at end expiration. Surfactant also enhances lung compliance, detoxifies inhaled gases, and coats particles that are inhaled.

13. **(C)** The units that are gas exchanging include the respiratory bronchioles, alveolar ducts, alveolar sacs, and alveoli. These are the most distal components of the tracheobronchial tree.

14. **(A)** A direct method for obtaining minute ventilation involves tidal volume measurements, which can be obtained at the bedside with hand-held devices. Minute ventilation ($\dot{V}_E$) equals tidal volume (V_T) multiplied by the respiratory rate (f), or $\dot{V}_E = V_T \times f$.

15. **(B)** Respiratory minute ventilation, or the volume of air inspired per minute, is equal to tidal volume times the respiratory rate.

16. **(C)** Minute alveolar ventilation ($\dot{V}_A$) can be calculated by subtracting the anatomic dead space volume (V_{Danat}) from the tidal volume (V_T) and then multiplying the result by the respiratory frequency (f), or:

$$\dot{V}_A = (V_T - V_{Danat}) \times f$$

Anatomic dead space is dependent on body size and can be estimated to approximate the individual's weight (e.g., a 190-lb person would have an estimated 190-ml anatomic dead space).

28. A 20-year-old female is admitted to the ICU in acute renal failure in a city whose atmospheric pressure is 760 mm Hg. She is breathing room air, and her blood gases indicate a Pa_{O_2} of 98 mm Hg and a Pa_{CO_2} of 34 mm Hg. What is her A-a gradient?

    A. 5 mm Hg.
    B. 9 mm Hg.
    C. 14 mm Hg.
    D. 20 mm Hg.

29. A normal A-a gradient in a young adult would be

    A. 8 mm Hg.
    B. 15 mm Hg.
    C. 20 mm Hg.
    D. 30 mm Hg.

30. The Pa_{O_2} is a measurement of

    A. Oxygen that combines with hemoglobin.
    B. The fraction of inspired oxygen.
    C. Oxygen dissolved in arterial plasma.
    D. Alveolar oxygen pressure.

31. The amount of oxygen transported in the circulation per minute is equal to

    A. Pa_{O_2} × the stroke volume.
    B. Arterial oxygen content × the cardiac output.
    C. Hemoglobin value × 98%.
    D. Heart rate × Pa_{O_2}.

Answers to Questions from page 4

17. (**B**) There is an inverse relationship between Pa_{CO_2} and alveolar ventilation when Pa_{CO_2} is outside normal limits. A Pa_{CO_2} within normal limits equates with adequate ventilation.

18. (**A**) Alveolar macrophages are activated in response to antigen stimulation of humoral and cell-mediated immune systems. Once macrophages phagocytize particles, the cilia transport them in mucus toward the glottis for removal. Some are eliminated through the pulmonary lymphatic system.

19. (**B**) The main muscle of quiet or resting respiration is the diaphragm. Accessory muscles, not usually used in quiet or resting respiration, include the pectoralis major, sternocleidomastoid, and intercostals.

20. (**D**) Expiration is usually a passive act that is predominantly due to lung recoil. When increased ventilation is necessary, the internal intercostal and abdominal muscles are called into action.

21. (**B**) Changes in the size of the thorax accomplished by respiratory muscles result in changes in intrathoracic pressures. When intrapulmonary pressure falls below atmospheric pressure, air enters the lung; when intrapulmonary pressure rises above atmospheric pressure, air exits the lung. The normally negative-to-atmospheric intrapleural pressure helps prevent lung collapse.

22. (**B**) *Compliance* refers to the distensibility of the lung. When compliance is high, the lung is more distensible. When compliance is low, the lung is stiff and resists distention.

32. The oxyhemoglobin dissociation (O_2-Hb) curve demonstrates the relationship between the Pa_{O_2} and

    A. Pa_{CO_2}.
    B. Renal function.
    C. FI_{O_2}.
    D. Oxygen saturation.

33. Before a patient who has suffered a respiratory arrest receives treatment, she would have an oxyhemoglobin dissociation (O_2-Hb) curve that

    A. Is normal.
    B. Shifts to the right.
    C. Shifts to the left.
    D. Assumes a flattened space.

34. Which of the following would cause the O_2-Hb curve to shift to the left?

    A. A pH of 7.30.
    B. An elevated temperature.
    C. An increased CPK level.
    D. A decreased level of 2,3 DPG.

35. The largest percentage of CO_2 carried in the blood is

    A. Carried as bicarbonate.
    B. Physically dissolved in the blood.
    C. Chemically combined with hemoglobin.
    D. Carried as ammonia.

36. The results from a mixed venous blood gas sample show your patient's mixed venous oxygen content ($C\bar{v}_{O_2}$) has fallen from 14 vol % to 7 vol %. Assuming that oxygen consumption has remained constant, these new data suggest

    A. That an arterial sample was inadvertently drawn.
    B. A recent elevation in Pa_{O_2}.
    C. A reduction in cardiac output.
    D. An elevation in functional hemoglobin.

Answers to Questions from page 5

23. **(C)** The medullary respiratory center coordinates the respiratory cycle, controls the rate and depth of respiration, responds to pH changes in cerebrospinal fluid, controls the diaphragm through phrenic nerve innervation, and responds to metabolic demands of the body by adjusting alveolar ventilation.

24. **(A)** There are thought to be two centers located in the pons that affect ventilation: the apneustic center, which is believed to stimulate inspiration, and the pneumotaxic center which is believed to stimulate expiration. The hypophysis is the pituitary body, whereas the cerebral cortex operates higher mental functions.

25. **(B)** Minute ventilation can be calculated by multiplying tidal volume (V_T) by respiratory rate (f).

26. **(A)** Alveolar ventilation is inversely related to Pa_{CO_2}. Normal Pa_{CO_2} range is 35–45 mm Hg; therefore, an elevated Pa_{CO_2} (50 mm Hg) indicates a decrease in alveolar ventilation.

27. **(A)** The alveolocapillary membrane is the structure through which diffusion of gases occurs. Because CO_2 is about 20 times more diffusible than O_2, damage to the membrane would significantly compromise the ability of O_2 to enter the blood more than it would affect the ability of CO_2 to exit the blood.

37. Which of the following statements regarding pulmonary circulation is *false?*

    A. The pulmonary circulation holds about 12% of the total blood volume at any one time.
    B. Compared with systemic circulation, the pulmonary circulation is a low-pressure, low-resistance system.
    C. In upright positions, the volume of blood in the pulmonary capillaries equals the stroke volume of the heart.
    D. The pulmonary arterial bed responds to alveolar hypoxia by vasodilation.

38. The most common cause of hypoxemia is

    A. Alveolar hypoventilation.
    B. Ventilation/perfusion mismatching.
    C. Low inspired O_2 tension.
    D. A decreased Pa_{CO_2}.

39. A patient on a mechanical ventilator has developed some areas of atelectasis. You would expect his $\dot{V}/\dot{Q}$ ratio to be

    A. Unmeasurable.
    B. Increased.
    C. Decreased.
    D. Unaffected.

40. Which of the following causes of hypoxemia can be corrected by administration of 100% O_2?

    A. Shunting.
    B. $\dot{V}/\dot{Q}$ mismatching.
    C. Atelectasis.
    D. ARDS.

41. For the blood pH to remain normal, the body attempts to maintain a ratio of bicarbonate to CO_2 of approximately

    A. 10:1.
    B. 20:1.
    C. 30:1.
    D. 50:1.

42. Which of the following parameters primarily reflects respiratory function?

    A. Pa_{CO_2}.
    B. CO_2 content.
    C. HCO_3^-.
    D Base excess.

Answers to Questions from page 6

28. (**B**) The A-a gradient is calculated by subtracting arterial oxygen pressure (Pa_{O_2}) from alveolar oxygen pressure (PA_{O_2}), or:

$$\text{A-a gradient} = PA_{O_2} - Pa_{O_2}$$

PA_{O_2} is equal to the pressure of inspired oxygen (PI_{O_2}) minus the Pa_{CO_2} divided by the respiratory quotient (0.8), or:

$$PA_{O_2} = PI_{O_2} - (Pa_{CO_2} \div 0.8)$$

The PI_{O_2} is equal to atmospheric pressure (P_B) minus 47, multiplied by the FI_{O_2}, or:

$$PI_{O_2} = (P_B - 47) \times FI_{O_2}$$

The whole equation can be stated thus:

$$\text{A-a gradient} = FI_{O_2} (P_B - 47) - (Pa_{CO_2} \div 0.8 - Pa_{O_2})$$

In the case described in the question, the equation would be:

$$.21 (760-47) - (34 \div 0.8) - 98 = 9$$

29. (**A**) The A-a gradient is a reflection of the difference between the pressure of oxygen in the alveoli and the pressure of oxygen in arterial blood. It is always a positive number and is less than 10 mm Hg in a young adult.

30. (**C**) The Pa_{O_2} is a measurement of oxygen dissolved in the arterial plasma and accounts for 3% of the total oxygen carried in the blood. 97% of the oxygen is carried in chemical combination with hemoglobin.

31. (**B**) The systemic oxygen transport (ml/min) is equal to the arterial oxygen content (ml/L) $\times$ the cardiac output (L/min). The arterial oxygen content (Ca_{O_2}) relates to the fact that each gram of hemoglobin can combine with a maximum of 1.34 ml of oxygen when it is fully saturated. The value obtained is called the O_2 capacity. Therefore, Ca_{O_2} is equal to the O_2 capacity $\times$ the oxygen saturation.

43. An elevation in Pa_{CO_2} (greater than 45 mm Hg) means that

    A. Hypoventilation is present.
    B. Hyperventilation is present.
    C. The kidneys are retaining H^+.
    D. The kidneys are excreting plasma proteins.

44. A patient with COPD will most likely demonstrate which of the following primary acid-base disturbances?

    A. Metabolic acidosis.
    B. Metabolic alkalosis.
    C. Respiratory acidosis.
    D. Respiratory alkalosis.

45. Which of the following findings supports metabolic alkalosis?

    A. Pa_{CO_2} of 40 mm Hg.
    B. pH of 7.32.
    C. Base excess of -4.
    D. HCO_3^- of 30 mEq/L.

46. The body attempts to compensate for respiratory alkalosis by

    A. Hyperventilating.
    B. Hypoventilating.
    C. Excreting HCO_3^- through the kidneys.
    D. Excreting H^+ through the kidneys.

47. Which of the following would you expect as compensation for diabetic ketoacidosis?

    A. Hyperventilation.
    B. Hypoventilation.
    C. Excretion of HCO_3^- through the kidneys.
    D. Excretion of H^+ through the kidneys.

48. A patient in the ICU has sepsis. Interpret her arterial blood gas data: FI_{O_2} 0.21; pH 7.33; P_{CO_2} 36; P_{O_2} 95; S_{O_2} 99.3%; HCO_3^- 18; B.E. -7.

    A. Uncompensated respiratory acidosis.
    B. Compensated respiratory alkalosis.
    C. Compensated metabolic alkalosis.
    D. Uncompensated metabolic acidosis.

Answers to Questions from page 7

32. (**D**) The oxyhemoglobin dissociation curve is an S-shaped curve that demonstrates the relationship between the oxygen saturation (Sa_{O_2}) and the Pa_{O_2}. It reflects hemoglobin's ability to bind O_2 at normal Pa_{O_2} levels and release it at lower Pa_{O_2} levels.

33. (**B**) This patient's oxyhemoglobin dissociation curve would demonstrate a shift to the right, where more O_2 is delivered and released to the tissues. Both the acidosis and the elevated Pa_{CO_2} that accompanies a respiratory arrest will cause the O_2-Hb curve to shift to the right.

34. (**D**) Since 2,3 diphosphoglycerate (2, 3 DPG) is an end product of metabolism that facilitates release of O_2 from hemoglobin at the tissues, decreased levels of 2, 3 DPG shift the O_2-Hb curve to the left. This shift results in decreased O_2 release to the tissues. Other factors that shift the curve to the left are alkalosis (increased pH), decreased Pa_{CO_2}, and decreased temperature.

35. (**A**) 60–70% of CO_2 in the body is found in the form of bicarbonate, produced by the following reaction:

$$CO_2 + H_2O \rightleftharpoons H_2CO_3 \rightleftharpoons H^+ + HCO_3^-$$

7–10% of CO_2 is physically dissolved in the blood (Pa_{CO_2}). The CO_2 that combines with hemoglobin (carbaminohemoglobin) accounts for about 30% of CO_2 in the blood.

36. (**C**) Two primary parameters influencing oxygenation are cardiac output and arterial oxygen content (Ca_{O_2}). If either parameter is reduced, tissue hypoxia can occur. Hypoxia results in greater tissue extraction of oxygen, which is reflected by a reduction in mixed venous oxygen content ($C\bar{v}_{O_2}$). The difference in arterial–mixed venous oxygen content (Ca-$\bar{v}_{O_2}$) reflects the amount of oxygen extracted by the tissues. Assuming that oxygen consumption remains constant, if the $C\bar{v}_{O_2}$ falls and the Ca-$\bar{v}_{O_2}$ rises, a reduction in cardiac output is suggested.

49. Interpret the following arterial blood gas data obtained from patient in the emergency room who has taken a drug overdose: FI_{O_2} 0.21; pH 7.35; P_{CO_2} 61; P_{O_2} 46; S_{O_2} 78%; HCO_3^- 33; B.E. +7.

    A. Normal acid-base balance.
    B. Compensated respiratory acidosis.
    C. Uncompensated respiratory alkalosis.
    D. Compensated metabolic acidosis.

50. On basis of the blood gas data given in question 49, which of the following would be most appropriate?

    A. Administer $NaHCO_3$.
    B. Start O_2 at 4 L per nasal cannula.
    C. Intubation and mechanical ventilation.
    D. No immediate action is necessary.

51. Interpret the following arterial blood gas data for an MI patient in the coronary care unit: FI_{O_2} 0.4; pH 7.42; P_{CO_2} 36; P_{O_2} 119; S_{O_2} 98%; HCO_3^- 23; B.E. −1.

    A. Normal acid-base balance.
    B. Compensated respiratory acidosis.
    C. Uncompensated metabolic alkalosis.
    D. Compensated metabolic acidosis.

52. Interpret the following arterial blood gas data for a woman 8 months pregnant: FI_{O_2} 0.21; pH 7.46; P_{CO_2} 29; P_{O_2} 84; S_{O_2} 98%; HCO_3^- 20; B.E. −3.

    A. Compensated respiratory acidosis.
    B. Uncompensated respiratory alkalosis.
    C. Compensated metabolic acidosis.
    D. Uncompensated metabolic alkalosis.

53. Which of the following may result in metabolic alkalosis?

    A. Cardiac arrest.
    B. Anxiety.
    C. Pulmonary embolus.
    D. Antacid administration.

Answers to Questions from page 8

37. (**D**) If alveolar hypoxia is diffuse, generalized vasoconstriction and pulmonary hypertension occur. Localized hypoxia results in localized vasoconstriction, which shunts blood away from poorly ventilated areas. This improves gas exchange and does not increase pulmonary arterial pressure.

38. (**B**) Ventilation/perfusion ($\dot{V}/\dot{Q}$) abnormalities, the most common cause of hypoxemia, are accompanied by an increased A-a gradient. Alveolar hypoventilation and low inspired O_2 tension are less common causes of hypoxemia.

39. (**C**) An individual with atelectasis would be expected to have a $\dot{V}/\dot{Q}$ ratio lower than the normal value of 0.8. In atelectasis, hypoxemia occurs owing to decreased ventilation secondary to alveolar collapse.

40. (**B**) Administration of 100% O_2 will correct $\dot{V}/\dot{Q}$ mismatching by washing all the nitrogen out and leaving O_2 and CO_2 in the alveoli. Shunting occurs because a portion of the venous blood does not participate in gas exchange. This condition cannot be corrected by 100% O_2 administration, because all blood doesn't interface with open alveoli, and hemoglobin cannot oversaturate to carry excess O_2. Atelectasis and adult respiratory distress syndrome (ARDS) are both accompanied by shunting.

41. (**B**) The Henderson-Hasselbach equation demonstrates the relationship between the pH, bicarbonate, and Pa_{CO_2}. The body attempts to maintain a relationship of HCO_3^- to CO_2 of about 20:1. This relationship results in a normal blood PH (7.35–7.45).

42. (**A**) The Pa_{CO_2} is a respiratory parameter. Abnormalities in Pa_{CO_2} will result in pH changes. HCO_3^- and base excess are nonrespiratory or renal parameters.

54. Obtaining a history is important in dealing with respiratory patients because

    A. It is the most unbiased component of assessment.
    B. It allows the examiner to dictate the plan of care to the patient.
    C. The examiner can control the interview to avoid dealing with unimportant emotional aspects of the patient.
    D. Childhood respiratory problems often correlate with adult respiratory diseases.

55. A respiratory patient complains of chest pain that is poorly localized in the center of his chest. Where does his pain most likely originate from?

    A. Visceral pleura.
    B. Parietal pleura.
    C. Intercostal muscles.
    D. Ribs.

56. When one is performing physical assessment techniques on the patient's chest, it is important to

    A. Auscultate prior to palpation to avoid alteration of your findings.
    B. Compare each side with the other.
    C. Assess the right and left sides of the chest independently because of anatomical differences.
    D. Choose a dark, quiet room.

57. You would expect increased vocal or tactile fremitus in a patient with

    A. Pneumonia.
    B. Pneumothorax.
    C. Emphysema.
    D. Pleural effusion.

58. When examining a patient, you note that he is barrel-chested. This can be

    A. A normal finding.
    B. A congenital condition.
    C. The result of hepatomegaly or cardiomegaly.
    D. The result of prolonged, generalized airway obstruction.

Answers to Questions from page 9

43. (**A**) As previously mentioned, the Pa_{CO_2} is a respiratory parameter. If Pa_{CO_2} is elevated, the individual is hypoventilating. If the Pa_{CO_2} is low (below 35 mm Hg), the individual is hyperventilating.

44. (**C**) Owing to the destruction of lung gas exchange tissue and to resultant $\dot{V}/\dot{Q}$ mismatching that accompany chronic obstructive pulmonary disease, an affected patient has a tendency to retain CO_2. Retention of CO_2 results in respiratory acidosis.

45. (**D**) Metabolic alkalosis occurs when HCO_3^- values are elevated. Base excess value will also rise (greater than $+2$). The pH demonstrates an alkalosis; that is, it will be greater than 7.45 (in the absence of compensation).

(**C**) Because the body cannot withstand excessive changes in pH, it responds physiologically to an acid-base irregularity by changes in the system not primarily affected. Compensation for respiratory alkalosis would result in excretion of HCO_3^- through the renal system. The respiratory system can compensate for metabolism acid-base disturbances much more rapidly than the renal system can compensate for respiratory acid-base disturbances.

47. (**A**) Diabetic ketoacidosis is a cause of metabolic acidosis. Compensation would occur in the respiratory system, in the form of attempts to reduce Pa_{CO_2} and thus raise the pH.

48. (**D**) The primary acid-base irregularity is metabolic acidosis, as evidenced by the acidotic pH and abnormally low levels of HCO_3^- and base excess. If compensation had occurred, we would expect to see a low Pa_{CO_2}, which would shift the pH back inside normal limits.

59. In percussion of the lungs, the sounds elicited over normal lung fields are

    A. Tympanitic.
    B. Resonant.
    C. Hyperresonant.
    D. Dull.

60. During auscultation of a patient's chest, you hear vesicular breath sounds on inspiration over the lung bases. You know this is

    A. Normal only on expiration.
    B. A sign of fluid in the airways.
    C. A normal finding.
    D. Normally heard only over the trachea.

61. Auscultation of an atelectatic right lower lobe will reveal

    A. Pleural friction rub.
    B. Decrease or absence of breath sounds.
    C. Increased tactile fremitus.
    D. Whispered pectoriloquy.

62. Percussion of an atelectatic lung reveals

    A. Resonance.
    B. Hyperresonance.
    C. Dullness.
    D. Tympany.

63. In making a respiratory assessment you ask an individual to say "EEEE" while you auscultate the chest. The sound you hear is "AAAA." What does this finding most likely indicate?

    A. You are listening over a pneumothorax.
    B. This is a normal finding.
    C. You are listening over a pleural effusion.
    D. There may be a pneumonia.

64. The total lung capacity is equal to

    A. V_T + IRV.
    B. ERV + RV.
    C. V_T + IRV + ERV + RV.
    D. V_T + IRV + ERV.

Answers to Questions from page 10

49. (**B**) This patient's primary acid-base problem is a respiratory acidosis. The pH is in the normal range but on the acidotic side of the median (7.40). The elevated P_{CO_2} confirms a respiratory acidosis. Because of the elevated HCO_3^- and the return of the pH to within normal limits, compensation can be confirmed.

50. (**C**) Owing to the marked hypoxemia and hypoventilation, this patient requires intubation and mechanical ventilation to raise the respiratory rate and deliver a higher FI_{O_2}. Because the primary acid-base problem is respiratory in nature, mechanical ventilation can correct the problem and possibly prevent the necessity of $NaHCO_3$ administration.

51. (**A**) This individual has normal acid-base balance. All parameters are within normal range (pH 7.35–7.45; P_{CO_2} 35–45; P_{O_2} 80–100; S_{O_2} 95% or greater; HCO_3^- 22–26; B.E. −2 to + 2).

52. (**B**) The primary acid-base problem is respiratory alkalosis secondary to hyperventilation. There are compensatory changes in the metabolic parameters; however, the pH is above normal limits. Respiratory alkalosis can sometimes occur during pregnancy.

53. (**D**) Ingestion of antacids may result in metabolic alkalosis. Cardiac arrest leads to metabolic acidosis because of lactic acid accumulation during anaerobic metabolism. Anxiety and pulmonary embolus result in hyperventilation, which can lead to respiratory alkalosis.

65. Which of the following statements regarding pulmonary function testing is *false*?

   A. Restrictive pulmonary disease usually results in decreased volumes and capacities.
   B. Patient values are compared with predicted values for age and sex.
   C. Increased pulmonary compliance indicates parenchymal disease.
   D. Obstructive pulmonary diseases usually result in decreased dynamic ventilatory function values.

66. The major nursing care objective for the respiratory patient is

   A. Effective oxygenation.
   B. Increased tidal volume.
   C. Improved inspiratory capacity.
   D. Increased A-a gradient.

67. In planning care for any respiratory patient, one would

   A. Administer prophylactic antibiotics.
   B. Provide large, nutritious meals.
   C. Encourage exercise to the initial stage of hypoxemia.
   D. Include a psychological assessment.

68. An observation consistent with complete airway obstruction is

   A. Loud "crowing" when attempting to speak.
   B. Inability to cough.
   C. Wheezes on auscultation.
   D. Gradual onset of respiratory difficulty.

69. When upper airway obstruction is suspected in the unconscious patient, the initial action is to

   A. Perform deep tracheal suction.
   B. Attempt mechanical ventilation.
   C. Tilt the head and lift the chin.
   D. Give upward abdominal thrusts.

70. Accumulation of secretions alters airway resistance. In the mechanically ventilated patient, this may be manifested by

   A. Increased pressure needed to deliver same tidal volume.
   B. Sudden rise in positive end expiratory pressure (PEEP).
   C. Decrease system pressure.
   D. Increased volume delivered with no additional pressure.

Answers to Questions from page 11

54. (D) There is a correlation between childhood respiratory problems and adult respiratory problems, which can be discerned from a history. The history is the component of assessment that is prone to bias; therefore, the examiner must remain objective. The examiner needs to take into account signs, symptoms, and emotional aspects of the patient when formulating a plan of care.

55. (A) Since the visceral pleura has no pain fibers, sensations originating here are usually central or substernal and poorly localized. Pain originating in the parietal pleura, intercostal muscles, or ribs is characteristically sharp and well-defined.

56. (B) Each side of the chest should be compared with the other side as a control, since the chest is usually bilaterally symmetrical. Palpation will alter auscultatory findings in the abdomen, not in the chest. A physical assessment should be performed in a quiet, well-lit room.

57. (A) Fremitus is a vibration that is heard or felt through the chest wall when the patient speaks. A condition associated with increased fremitus is pneumonia. Pneumothorax, emphysema, and pleural effusion interfere with the transmission of sound through the chest, resulting in diminished fremitus.

58. (D) An individual with prolonged, generalized airway obstruction can have an increased AP diameter, resulting in a chest that resembles a barrel. Emphysema patients frequently develop barrel chest.

71. To prevent complications that may arise from tracheobronchial suctioning, one should

    A. Keep the patient in a supine position.
    B. Administer atropine if bradycardia occurs.
    C. Hyperoxygenate the patient with 100% oxygen.
    D. Insert the catheter no more than 5 inches.

72. Mouth-to-mouth ventilation may be enhanced by

    A. Inserting a nasopharyngeal airway.
    B. Inserting an oropharyngeal airway.
    C. Removing the patient's dentures.
    D. Performing frequent gastric decompression.

73. An advantage of bag-valve-mask devices is that they

    A. Deliver larger tidal volumes than mouth-to-mouth ventilation.
    B. Prevent gastric distention.
    C. May be used successfully by inexperienced rescuers.
    D. Provide an indication of lung compliance.

74. A disadvantage of the esophageal obturator airway (EOA) is that

    A. Its removal usually evokes regurgitation.
    B. Its use is usually accompanied by gastric distention.
    C. It must be removed for endotracheal intubation.
    D. It requires a high tracheal cuff pressure.

75. Assessment techniques useful in ascertaining proper endotracheal tube placement include all except

    A. Inspection.
    B. Palpation.
    C. Percussion.
    D. Auscultation.

Answers to Questions from page 12

59. (B) Normal lung fields produce resonance. When there is an increase in air, you may elicit hyperresonance or tympany. When there is a solid mass or an increase in fluid, you may elicit dullness or flatness.

60. (C) Vesicular breath sounds are soft sounds normally heard over lung fields. They are heard primarily on inspiration.

61. (B) Atelectasis is associated with a decrease or absence of vesicular breath sounds, and diminution or absence of tactile fremitus.

62. (C) When solid tissue or fluid replaces air-filled lung areas, dullness is heard.

63. (D) Egophony is the voice sound that translates a spoken "EEEE" to an auscultated "AAAA." This is heard over parts of the lung where air has been replaced by solid or liquid. With a pneumothorax or pleural effusion, voice sounds are significantly diminished. You may detect egophony immediately above a pleural effusion.

64. (C) The total lung capacity (TLC) is the total amount of gas contained in the lung at the end of a maximal inspiration. This would include the tidal volume (V_T), the inspiratory reserve volume (IRC), the expiratory reserve volume (ERV), and the residual volume (RV). The inspiratory capacity (IC) is equal to the V_T plus the IRV. The functional residual capacity (FRC) is equal to the ERV plus the RV. The vital capacity (VC) is equal to the V_T plus the IRV plus the ERV.

76. Endotracheal tube cuff pressure should never exceed

   A. 10 mm Hg.
   B. 30 mm Hg.
   C. 45 mm Hg.
   D. 60 mm Hg.

77. Nursing care for the patient with tracheal intubation utilizing a low pressure cuff should include

   A. Routine cuff deflation to prevent necrosis.
   B. Routine measurement of cuff pressure.
   C. Maintaining 10 ml of air in the cuff.
   D. Deflation of cuff during inspiration.

78. Nursing care in the immediate postextubation period should include all of the following measures except

   A. Encouraging deep breathing.
   B. Auscultating for stridor.
   C. Evaluation of pharyngeal reflexes.
   D. Deep pharyngeal suctioning.

79. The observation that best indicates intolerance to extubation is

   A. Dyspnea.
   B. Hyperalertness.
   C. Throat pain.
   D. Tachycardia.

80. One indication that the cuff on a tracheostomy tube is deflated is

   A. Ineffective cough.
   B. Dysphagia.
   C. Vocal sounds.
   D. Secretions oozing from incision site.

81. When one is conducting a dye test, the immediate presence of methylene blue in tracheal aspirate could indicate

   A. Peristomal skin breakdown.
   B. Barotrauma.
   C. Esophageal varices.
   D. Tracheoesophageal fistula.

Answers to Questions from page 13

65. (C) Parenchymal disease, particularly infiltrative or interstitial disease, is indicated by decreased pulmonary compliance. In emphysema there is an increase in compliance.

66. (A) Effective oxygenation is achieved when all components of respiration are functional. Although improvement in any single component—such as tidal volume, alveolar ventilation, oxygen transport, or oxygen uptake—may enhance oxygenation, no one component can produce effective oxygenation. Intervention may deal with any or all components in an attempt to achieve the basic goal of effective oxygenation.

67. (D) Psychological support is an integral part of care for any respiratory patient; thus, care planning should always include psychological assessment. Although helpful in some situations, prophylactic antibiotics would not be routinely used in all pulmonary patients. Other important aspects of care include rest and adequate nutrition. Unnecessary oxygen-consuming activities, such as digestion of large meals and physical exertion, should be avoided.

68. (B) In complete airway obstruction, there is no passage of air, so all speech and breath sounds are absent. Complete airway obstruction is generally acute.

69. (C) The head-tilt, chin-lift maneuver lifts the tongue from the posterior pharynx to allow for free passage of air. This must be accomplished before artificial ventilation can be effective. Abdominal thrusts should be utilized when less aggressive techniques fail. Deep tracheal suction should be avoided, in order to prevent further lodging of any upper airway foreign body.

70. (A) Pressure changes on the ventilator reflect changes in compliance. Accumulated secretions decrease compliance; therefore, there is an increase in the amount of pressure necessary to deliver a specified volume.

82. Which of the following signs would be considered most serious in the early post-extubation period?

    A. Hoarseness.
    B. Inspiratory stridor.
    C. Decreased ability to swallow liquids.
    D. Sore throat.

83. A patient receiving mechanical ventilation receives augmentation for eight spontaneous breaths and four ventilator-initiated breaths within 1 minute. The mode of ventilation is

    A. Assisted.
    B. Controlled.
    C. PEEP.
    D. Assist-control.

84. In the presence of a ruptured balloon on an endotracheal tube, continuous inspiration may be delivered by which mode of mechanical ventilation?

    A. Pressure-cycled.
    B. Volume-cycled.
    C. Time-cycled.
    D. Flow-cycled.

85. The mode of mechanical ventilation most effective for patients with copious pulmonary secretions would be

    A. Pressure-cycled.
    B. Volume-cycled.
    C. Time-cycled.
    D. Flow-cycled.

86. Periodic sigh ventilations serve to

    A. Prevent microatelectasis.
    B. Elevate Pa_{O_2}
    C. Reduce Pa_{O_2}.
    D. Increase humidification.

87. Inadequate airway humidification may be indicated by

    A. Copious watery secretions.
    B. Scant thick secretions.
    C. Decreased core body temperature.
    D. Decreased airway pressure.

Answers to Questions from page 14

71. (**C**) Hyperoxygenation is utilized to prevent hypoxemia that is due to suctioning. It should be used for most patients requiring suctioning, even those not on a ventilator. Changes in heart rate during suctioning suggest hypoxemia and should be managed by immediate reestablishment of ventilation and oxygenation.

72. (**B**) If available, the oropharyngeal airway will assist in pathway patency. Nasopharyngeal airways would be helpful in mouth-to-nose ventilation but would be of no value in mouth-to-mouth ventilation. Dentures left in place assist in achieving an adequate seal. Owing to the risk of regurgitation, gastric decompression should be utilized only when necessary.

73. (**D**) The operator of a bag-valve-mask device is provided with a gross indication of lung compliance by the amount of pressure needed to effect ventilation. Because of difficulty in achieving an adequate seal, the device often delivers a smaller tidal volume than mouth-to-mouth ventilation.

74. (**A**) The EOA is a blind-ended tube that utilizes an inflatable cuff to occlude the esophagus. Endotracheal intubation may be accomplished with the EOA in place. Regurgitation should be anticipated upon removal of the EOA.

75. (**C**) Although percussion is a useful respiratory assessment technique, it is of no value in ascertaining proper tube placement. Inspection and palpation of symmetrical chest wall movement and auscultation for equal breath sounds are routine techniques to evaluate placement of the tube immediately upon its insertion.

88. Increasing the negative force required to trigger mechanical augmentation may be accomplished by decreasing the

    A. Rate.
    B. Sigh volume.
    C. PEEP.
    D. Sensitivity.

89. Upon institution of positive pressure ventilation, the nurse should be alert for which potential hemodynamic response?

    A. Hypotension.
    B. Hypertension.
    C. Increased cardiac output.
    D. Bradycardia.

90. Hypotension associated with positive pressure ventilation may be decreased by

    A. FI_{O_2} increase.
    B. Preload reduction.
    C. External cardiac massage.
    D. Trendelenburg position.

91. Pneumothorax may be one complication of positive pressure ventilation. One sign of pneumothorax is

    A. Hemoptysis.
    B. Dull, aching chest pain.
    C. Asymmetrical chest movement.
    D. Decreased inspiratory pressures.

92. One factor that may preclude ventilator independence is

    A. Psychological dependence.
    B. Increased FRC.
    C. Intrapulmonary shunting of 8% on ventilator.
    D. Dead space–tidal volume ratio of 40%.

93. One potential complication of humidification is

    A. Fluid overload.
    B. Thickened secretions.
    C. Decreased A-a gradient.
    D. Decreased V_D/V_T ratios.

94. Gastric dilatation in the mechanically ventilated patient is usually caused by

    A. Immobility.
    B. Hypervolemia.
    C. Swallowed air.
    D. Leaks in the endotracheal tube cuff.

Answers to Questions from page 15

76. **(B)** Cuff pressure should never exceed 25–30 mm Hg and should be maintained at the lowest pressure possible to establish an adequate seal during positive pressure ventilation. Pressures greater than 25–30 mm Hg occlude arterial-capillary blood flow. Venous blood flow is compromised at even lower pressures.

77. **(B)** Cuff pressure should be measured in every patient any time the cuff is reinflated as well as routinely not less than every 8 hours. Air need be injected only until there is no audible leak over the trachea. Deflation of the cuff should be performed only during expiration, so that secretions pooled above the cuff will be propelled to the oropharynx by expiration.

78. **(D)** Deep pharyngeal suctioning would increase the risk of laryngospasm, which is one of the more common complications of the early post-extubation period.

79. **(A)** Throat pain is expected and normal after intubation. Hyperalertness and tachycardia may suggest intolerance but may also be due to the anxiety associated with extubation. Dyspnea is the most sensitive marker of respiratory effort.

80. **(C)** When the cuff of an appropriately fitted tracheostomy tube is inflated, air does not pass through the larynx, and the patient is aphonic. Vocal sounds indicate that air is passing around the cuff through the larynx.

81. **(D)** The methylene blue dye test involves having the patient drink a dye solution. It is used to confirm a suspicion of tracheoesophageal (T-E) fistula. When a T-E fistula is present, the dye solution will immediately be present in significant quantity in the trachea.

95. Bowel sound assessment for adynamic ileus in the respiratory patient should include auscultation for at least

    A. 30 seconds.
    B. 1 minute.
    C. 2 minutes.
    D. 5 minutes.

96. The mechanically ventilated patient who becomes combative should be immediately evaluated for

    A. Chest pain.
    B. Psychosis.
    C. Hypoxia.
    D. Sensory deprivation.

97. You note a mechanically ventilated patient to be extremely agitated. The pressure alarm sounds with each inspiration. An appropriate initial nursing response would be to

    A. Increase the respiratory rate.
    B. Increase the pressure limit.
    C. Decrease the tidal volume.
    D. Ventilate with a self-inflating bag.

98. Which of the following would be most predictive of successful weaning from a mechanical ventilator?

    A. Resting minute volume of 15 L.
    B. A-a gradient of 12 mm Hg.
    C. Inspiratory pressure of -10cm H_2O pressure.
    D. Resting minute ventilation equal to maximum voluntary ventilation.

99. During the first 15 minutes of ventilator independence, which would be most indicative of intolerance?

    A. Mild elevation in blood pressure.
    B. Mild diaphoresis.
    C. Slight increase in heart rate.
    D. Onset of ventricular ectopy.

100. During intermittent mandatory ventilation (IMV), the ventilator

    A. Cycles on each inspiratory effort by the patient.
    B. Slightly augments each spontaneous breath.
    C. Delivers a preset number of breaths per minute.
    D. Requires a separate oxygen source for spontaneous breaths.

82. (**B**) Prolonged intubation frequently results in sore throat, hoarseness, and less effective protective laryngeal reflexes. These symptoms usually disappear during the first week. Inspiratory stridor in early post-extubation period signals glottic edema, which could progress to complete airway obstruction.

83. (**D**) The assist-control mode may be set to deliver a minimum number of respirations per minute, augment spontaneous respirations, and initiate respirations on demand.

84. (**A**) Pressure-cycled ventilators maintain the inspiratory phase until a preset airway pressure is achieved. Escape of air around the cuff may preclude the rise in pressure needed to terminate the inspiratory phase.

85. (**B**) Secretions may reduce airway compliance, so that a greater pressure is needed to deliver the preset volume.

86. (**A**) Periodic sigh ventilations are believed to prevent microatelectasis caused by constant volume ventilation.

87. (**B**) Drying of secretions indicates decreased humidity. Thick, immobile secretions would increase airway pressure.

101. Essential to effective chest physiotherapy is

    A. Patient's ability to tolerate head-down position.
    B. Cardiac monitoring.
    C. Effective cough or suction.
    D. Use of aerosol bronchodilators.

102. Which action should follow therapeutic drainage of the affected lung in a patient with unilateral pneumonia?

    A. Return patient to semi-Fowler's position.
    B. Drain the opposite lung.
    C. Culture secretions coughed up.
    D. Obtain arterial blood gases.

103. Early symptoms of hypoxia include

    A. Confusion.
    B. Cyanosis.
    C. Polycythemia.
    D. Pupillary changes.

104. A COPD patient would respond to high concentrations of oxygen by

    A. An increase in myocardial work.
    B. A decrease in ventilatory work.
    C. No change in ventilatory work.
    D. A decrease in alveolar oxygen tension.

105. One disadvantage of high-flow oxygen delivery systems is that they

    A. Do not provide the full inspired volume of air.
    B. Are incapable of delivering low oxygen concentrations.
    C. Are generally uncomfortable for patients.
    D. Have no mechanism to control gas humidity.

106. Retrolental fibroplasia, a complication of oxygen therapy, is associated with a

    A. Pa_{CO_2} of less than 20 mm Hg.
    B. Pa_{CO_2} of greater than 60 mm Hg.
    C. Pa_{O_2} of less than 60 mm Hg.
    D. Pa_{O_2} of greater than 100 mm Hg.

Answers to Questions from page 17

88. (**D**) Sensitivity setting delineates the "trigger" for sensing the patient's intrinsic inspiratory effect. Decreasing the sensitivity increases the force needed to trigger the ventilator.

89. (**A**) Positive pressure ventilation may result in some decrease in venous return. This decrease creates the potential for hypotension, especially in the critically ill patient with poor cardiovascular reserves.

90. (**D**) Because hypotension related to positive ventilation is frequently transient, the Trendelenburg position may be used. In persistent hypotension, medical management, such as preload manipulation through administration of fluids, may be required.

91. (**C**) Symptoms of pneumothorax vary, depending on its size and type. Unilateral chest movement and increased inspiratory pressures are frequently seen. Accompanying chest pain is more commonly sharp and pleuritic.

92. (**A**) Psychological dependence is a common cause of weaning difficulty in the absence of physiological indicators. $\dot{Q}S/\dot{Q}T$ of less than 20% on the ventilator is compatible with ventilator independence.

93. (**A**) Fluid overload may result from retention of inspired water vapor.

94. (**C**) Gastric dilatation commonly occurs because of a tendency to swallow air with an artificial airway in place.

107. In which instance would oxygen toxicity be of greatest concern?

    A. 35% oxygen for 3 days; pre-existing pulmonary disease.
    B. 70% oxygen for 3 days.
    C. 35% oxygen for 7 days.
    D. 100% oxygen for 2 hours; respiratory distress.

108. Many early symptoms of oxygen toxicity are related to

    A. Suppression of respiratory drive.
    B. Alveolar distention.
    C. Paralysis of respiratory muscles.
    D. Irritation of respiratory passages.

109. The oxygen delivery mask capable of delivering the highest oxygen concentration is the

    A. Simple.
    B. Venturi.
    C. Partial rebreathing.
    D. Nonrebreathing.

110. The nonrebreathing mask is capable of high concentrations of oxygen because of

    A. A reservoir bag.
    B. A leakproof face seal.
    C. A two-way valve.
    D. Small exhalation ports.

111. Basic to the proper function of any oxygen mask is

    A. A flow rate less than 6 L/min.
    B. An oxygen reservoir bag.
    C. A proper fit.
    D. A consistent ventilatory pattern.

112. If 6 inches of dead space were added to each exhalation port of a Venturi mask utilizing a high flow rate, the result would be

    A. Increased oxygen concentration in inspired air.
    B. Increased carbon dioxide concentration in inspired air.
    C. Varied with depth of inspiration.
    D. No significant change.

Answers to Questions from page 18

95. (**C**) Auscultation for bowel sounds should continue for a minimum of 2 minutes before their absence is diagnosed. Frequency of bowel sounds varies from five to 34 times per minute. Auscultation for 2 minutes should avoid failure to detect hypoactive bowel sounds.

96. (**C**) Hypoxia should be immediately considered as the cause of any change in personality or sensorium in the mechanically ventilated patient.

97. (**D**) When the mechanically ventilated patient "fights" the ventilator, adequate ventilation should be assured before adjustments are made on the ventilator. Manually ventilating the patient with a self-inflating bag allows an estimate of airway resistance. Other appropriate maneuvers include assessment for hypoxia, psychological support, suctioning, and validation of ventilator function.

98. (**B**) Successful weaning from mechanical ventilation is more likely if specific respiratory parameters (such as resting minute volume, inspiratory and expiratory pressures, arterial blood gases, tidal volume, vital capacity, and maximum voluntary effort) are within appropriate ranges. Specific predictors of successful weaning are (1) resting minute volume less than 10 L, (2) maximum voluntary ventilation that is twice the resting volume, (3) inspiratory force of at least -20 cm H_2O, and (4) an A-a gradient of less than 15 mm Hg.

99. (**D**) Due to the work of spontaneous respiration, mild increases in heart rate and blood pressure are often seen. Mild diaphoresis is also common. New onset of ventricular ectopy may result from hypoxia.

100. (**C**) IMV delivers a preset number of breaths per minute. Between ventilations, the ventilator serves as an oxygen reservoir, providing a specified O_2 concentration for spontaneous breaths. Ventilator cycles per minute may be slowly decreased as weaning progresses.

113. Oxygen delivery via nasal cannula would be least effective in the presence of

   A. Slow, shallow breathing pattern.
   B. Mouth breathing.
   C. Swollen nasal passages.
   D. COPD.

114. Hyperbaric oxygenation results in

   A. Increased $F_{I_{O_2}}$.
   B. Increased amount of dissolved oxygen in plasma.
   C. Decreased risk of oxygen toxicity.
   D. Increased surfactant production.

115. Positive end expiratory pressure (PEEP) is added in order to

   A. Decrease compliance.
   B. Avoid development of pneumothorax.
   C. Prevent alveolar collapse at end expiration.
   D. Equalize inspiratory/expiratory ratio.

116. One observation that indicates intolerance to PEEP is

   A. Rales.
   B. Hypertension.
   C. Intercostal chest discomfort.
   D. Decreased cardiac output.

117. The patient receiving PEEP might be expected to experience

   A. Intercostal chest discomfort.
   B. Substernal chest pain.
   C. Hemoptysis.
   D. Confusion.

118. A major goal of PEEP therapy is to accomplish

   A. Full inflation of the lung.
   B. A prolonged expiratory phase.
   C. Complete exhalation.
   D. A lower $F_{I_{O_2}}$.

119. The hemodynamic effect of morphine sulfate is

   A. Increased preload.
   B. Reduced afterload.
   C. Increased systemic vascular resistance.
   D. Increased PCWP.

Answers to Questions from page 19

101. **(C)** One goal of physiotherapy is the mobilization of secretions to an area where they can be removed via cough or suction. Head-down position utilizes gravity to facilitate upward movement of secretions. When head-down position cannot be tolerated, physiotherapy may be effective because of the action of pulmonary cilia, which escalate secretions upward.

102. **(B)** In unilateral disease, mobilization of secretions may be a source of contamination to the other lung. Therefore, therapeutic drainage should be followed by prophylactic drainage of the opposite lung.

103. **(A)** Because the brain is one of the organs most sensitive to hypoxia, altered mental status is seen very early. Cyanosis and pupillary changes may be seen later, depending on the severity of the hypoxia. Polycythemia is a compensatory response to chronic hypoxia.

104. **(B)** The chronically hypercarbic patient breathes only hard enough to maintain his usual state of oxygenation. Administration of high levels of oxygen will elevate alveolar oxygen levels. Because he works only hard enough to maintain usual oxygenation, he will decrease ventilatory and myocardial workload in the presence of elevated alveolar tension.

105. **(C)** High-flow oxygen delivery devices deliver a fast flow of a specific blend of room air and oxygen. Because the full inspired volume is supplied by the device, consistent temperature, humidity, and $F_{I_{O_2}}$ may be maintained, even in the presence of ventilatory variation, when appropriate flow rates are provided. These devices are, however, costly and uncomfortable for patients.

106. **(D)** An arterial P_{O_2} greater than 100 mm Hg is associated with retrolental fibroplasia. This is the oxygen level that the retinal vessels are actually exposed to.

120. Advantages of the depolarizing muscle relaxant succinylcholine include

    A. Rapid onset.
    B. Reversibility.
    C. Long duration.
    D. Sedative effect.

121. One disadvantage of bronchodilators is

    A. Limited routes of administration.
    B. Diuretic effect.
    C. Increased myocardial oxygen consumption.
    D. C.N.S. depression.

122. A patient is admitted to the intensive care unit in acute respiratory failure secondary to Guillain-Barré syndrome. Arterial blood gases will show

    A. An elevated Pa_{O_2} and an elevated Pa_{CO_2}.
    B. An elevated Pa_{O_2} and a decreased Pa_{CO_2}.
    C. A decreased Pa_{O_2} and elevated Pa_{CO_2}.
    D. A decreased Pa_{O_2} and a decreased Pa_{CO_2}.

123. When an individual is at rest and breathing room air, one parameter that defines acute respiratory failure is

    A. A Pa_{O_2} greater than 80 mm Hg.
    B. A Pa_{O_2} less than 60 mm Hg.
    C. A bicarbonate of 22–26 mEq/L.
    D. A base excess of -2 to $+2$.

124. Acute respiratory failure secondary to chronic obstructive pulmonary disease is characterized by

    A. The inability of the lungs to excrete CO_2 normally.
    B. An increase in extravascular lung water.
    C. The inability of the neuromuscular apparatus to ventilate the lungs.
    D. The inability of the lungs to retain CO_2 normally.

125. Which of the following *would not* be expected in a patient with hypercapnia coupled with acidemia?

    A. Headache.
    B. Unusual lucidity.
    C. Asterixis.
    D. Irritability.

Answers to Questions from page 20

107. **(B)** Administration of high concentrations (greater than 40%) of oxygen may result in oxygen toxicity. Toxicity is rarely seen with FI_{O_2} below 40%, even with prolonged use. Administration of 100% O_2 for brief periods is not contraindicated in emergency situations. Pre-existing pulmonary disease has not been correlated with increased risk of oxygen toxicity.

108. **(D)** Early signs of oxygen toxicity, such as substernal distress, sore throat, coughing, and restlessness, result from irritation of respiratory passages. This irritation may be due, in part, to decreased surfactant production.

109. **(D)** Nonrebreathing masks are capable of delivering oxygen concentrations of 90–100% when used properly.

110. **(A)** The nonrebreathing mask can deliver high oxygen concentrations because all of inspired volume is provided from the oxygen-rich reservoir bag. The flow rate should be adequate to fill the reservoir, which partially deflates on inspiration. The one-way valve seals the reservoir, forcing exhaled air out exhalation ports, while the oxygen source refills the reservoir.

111. **(C)** Masks generally come in only one adult size. Snug fit is essential to prevent the inhalation of air or the escape of oxygen around the mask. The flow rate should never be less than 6 L/min, in order to assure complete washing out of expired air from the mask.

112. **(A)** In the presence of high flow rate, the expired gas would be "washed" from the dead space, causing it to serve as a reservoir, thus increasing inspired oxygen concentration.

126. Arterial blood gases of patients with chronic hypoxemia and hypercapnia demonstrate

    A. A relatively normal pH.
    B. An alkaline pH.
    C. A decrease in blood buffers.
    D. A normal oxygen saturation.

127. Which of the following nursing implementations would be questionable for a patient in acute respiratory failure?

    A. Endotracheal intubation.
    B. Oxygen administration.
    C. Theophylline administration.
    D. Use of a rebreathing mask.

128. Which of the following statements regarding the pathophysiology of acute respiratory distress syndrome (ARDS) is *true*?

    A. There is decreased capillary permeability.
    B. There is damage to type II pneumocytes with a decrease of surfactant.
    C. There is a decrease in surface tension.
    D. There is a high Pa_{O_2}.

129. In evaluating the pulmonary function of a patient with ARDS, you would expect

    A. A reduced functional residual capacity (FRC).
    B. An increased lung compliance.
    C. A decreased A-a gradient.
    D. No intrapulmonary shunting.

130. In formulating a nursing plan to care for a patient with ARDS, your primary goals would be to

    A. Improve nutritional status and decrease pulmonary compliance.
    B. Hydrate the patient aggressively, in order to promote renal function, and to administer prophylactic antibiotics.
    C. Decrease blood pressure and increase Pa_{CO_2}.
    D. Improve oxygenation and pulmonary function.

Answers to Questions from page 21

113. (**C**) Patent nasal passages are essential for successful use of nasal cannula. Mouth breathing does not affect $F_{I_{O_2}}$, because the oropharynx serves as an anatomic reservoir.

114. (**B**) Hyperbaric oxygen markedly increases the amount of oxygen dissolved in plasma. The greater the delivery pressure, the more rapid the onset of oxygen toxicity symptoms.

115. (**C**) PEEP maintains a preset positive pressure in the alveoli at the end of expiration, serving to prevent or minimize alveolar collapse. This increases the FRC (functional residual capacity) and reduces the shunt effect of collapsed alveoli.

116. (**D**) Intolerance to PEEP is indicated by symptoms of decreased venous return.

117. (**A**) PEEP, especially at high levels, frequently produces intercostal chest discomfort.

118. (**D**) Increasing FRC (functional residual capacity) decreases the work of breathing and alveolar shunting. An acceptable Pa_{O_2} may be achieved at a lower $F_{I_{O_2}}$ than would be possible without PEEP.

119. (**B**) A sympatholytic action causes venous pooling, resulting in decreases in preload, SVR, and afterload.

131. Physiologic changes associated with COPD include

    A. Decreased airflow resistance on expiration.
    B. Even distribution of ventilation.
    C. Unchanged alveolar oxygenation.
    D. Increasing ventilation-perfusion disparity.

132. The incidence of COPD is frequently associated with

    A. Chronic bronchial irritation.
    B. Cool climate.
    C. Rural dwelling.
    D. Influenza vaccinations.

133. A common finding of chest auscultation of a patient with emphysema is

    A. Inspiratory wheezes.
    B. Increased vesicular breath sounds.
    C. Distant breath sounds.
    D. Pleural friction rub.

134. Physical findings consistent with COPD include all of the following *except*

    A. Increased AP chest diameter.
    B. Expiratory wheeze at end of forced expiration.
    C. Slow, deep respirations.
    D. Decreased diaphragmatic excursion.

135. One compensatory response of severe COPD is

    A. Diaphragmatic flattening.
    B. Bullae formation.
    C. Polycythemia.
    D. Goblet-cell hyperplasia.

136. The COPD patient is at an increased risk for pulmonary embolus because of

    A. Decreased activity.
    B. Increased viscosity of blood.
    C. Alveolar degeneration.
    D. Sluggish pulmonary circulation.

Answers to Questions from page 22

120. (**A**) The onset of action of succinylocholine occurs within 10 seconds; its effect is of short duration and irreversible.

121. (**C**) Most bronchodilators cause tachycardia and palpitations, thus increasing myocardial oxygen consumption. Bronchodilators, depending on type, may be administered by inhalation, orally, parenterally, or rectally.

122. (**C**) The inability of the neuromuscular apparatus to ventilate the lungs leads to a reduced arterial oxygen tension and an increased arterial carbon dioxide tension.

123. (**B**) When a patient is at rest and breathing room air, acute respiratory failure is defined by a Pa_{O_2} of less than 60 mm Hg. Normal Pa_{O_2} range is 80–100 mm Hg. Normal range for bicarbonate is 22–26 mEq/L, and normal range for base excess is -2 to $+2$. Both bicarbonate and base excess are generally considered nonrespiratory parameters of arterial blood gases but may change during the body's attempt to compensate for acid-base irregularities.

124. (**A**) In chronic obstructive disease, the lungs are frequently unable to excrete CO_2 normally. Patients with cardiogenic or noncardiogenic pulmonary edema and other parenchymal infiltrates may develop acute respiratory failure owing to an increase in extravascular lung water. Patients with neuromuscular diseases, chest wall diseases, or drug overdoses may develop acute respiratory failure owing to the inability of the neuromuscular apparatus to ventilate the lungs.

125. (**B**) Patients with hypercapnia coupled with acidemia will exhibit confusion because of decreased Pa_{O_2} and increased Pa_{CO_2}.

137. When an asthmatic patient encounters various irritating stimuli, the bronchial tree

   A. Becomes hyperreactive.
   B. Is unaffected.
   C. Discourages mucus production.
   D. Enlarges.

138. Which of the following signs and symptoms of asthma is seen early and is classically associated with the condition?

   A. Physical exhaustion.
   B. Dehydration.
   C. Wheezing.
   D. Tachypnea.

139. Which of the following nursing actions would be inappropriate for an asthmatic patient?

   A. Restrict fluid intake.
   B. Administer bronchodilators.
   C. Institute cardiac monitoring for dysrhythmias.
   D. Provide psychological support.

140. A common symptom of pulmonary embolus is

   A. Dyspnea.
   B. Hypotension.
   C. Increased P_{CO_2}.
   D. Chest pain.

141. When chest pain is associated with pulmonary embolus, it often

   A. Is dull and aching.
   B. Subsides with rest.
   C. Is aggravated by breathing.
   D. Has a gradual onset.

142. Streptokinase acts to restore normal circulation by

   A. Clot lysis.
   B. Relaxation of vasospasms.
   C. Vasodilation.
   D. Collateral formation.

143. Flail chest may be described as

   A. Abnormal thoracic contour secondary to COPD.
   B. Instability of chest wall due to rib fractures.
   C. Convexity of the anterior chest.
   D. Costal angle greater than 45 degrees.

Answers to Questions from page 23

126. (A) In the acute stages of hypoxemia and hypercapnia, particularly when accompanied by CHF, arterial pH reflects acidemia because of lactic acid production during anaerobic metabolism. As this process continues, the kidneys attempt to compensate for the acidosis by reabsorbing excess blood buffers. This increase in alkalinity tends to offset the acidosis and leads to a relatively normal pH. Hypoxemia and resulting acidosis cause a shift to the right of the oxygen-hemoglobin dissociation curve, leading to a decreased oxygen saturation.

127. (D) The use of a rebreathing mask in a patient with acute respiratory failure would be questionable because of the tendency of such a patient for hypercapnia. Patients in acute respiratory failure require oxgen administration to offset the hypoxemia. This is frequently best accomplished through intubation and mechanical ventilation. Theophylline will effect smooth muscle relaxation to dilate the bronchial tree.

128. (B) In ARDS, damage to type II pneumocytes results in decreased production of surfactant, which causes surface tension to increase. There is increased capillary permeability, leading to interstitial and alveolar edema. This combination of events lead to hypoxemia (low Pa_{O_2}).

129. (A) Patients with ARDS have a reduced FRC because of the interstitial and alveolar edema and microatelectasis that are associated with increased alveolar-capillary permeability. They will also have reduced compliance, increased A-a gradient, and a large right-to-left shunt.

130. (D) Your goals would be to increase Pa_{O_2} and improve pulmonary function by increasing compliance and FRC. Fluid administration to ARDS patients should be judicious and guided by hemodynamic parameters. ARDS patients frequently present with hypotension and usually are not hypercapnic initially.

144. Following a penetrating injury to the left chest, a patient is noted to have asymmetrical chest wall movement, dyspnea, and tracheal deviation to the right. These findings are characteristic of a

    A. Tension pneumothorax.
    B. Hemothorax.
    C. Rupture of the diaphragm.
    D. Flail chest.

145. Following severe blunt chest trauma sustained in an automobile accident, the patient complains of difficulty breathing and severe sharp chest pain. Nursing assessment reveals bounding carotid and brachial pulses and nonpalpable femoral pulses. This information leads the nurse to suspect

    A. Myocardial infarction.
    B. Cardiac tamponade.
    C. Aortic rupture.
    D. Rib fractures.

146. In which instance would a patient be at a greater risk of aspiration?

    A. Peptic ulcer disease.
    B. ET tube in place.
    C. Continuous enteral feedings via mercury-tipped feeding tube.
    D. Immediately post-extubation after long intubation.

147. Aspiration of water decreases compliance by altering

    A. Pulmonary blood flow.
    B. Length of expiration.
    C. Surfactant production.
    D. Oxygen concentration in inspired air.

148. Hemodilution and hypervolemia occur as a result of which type of drowning?

    A. Salt-water drowning.
    B. Fresh-water drowning.
    C. "Dry" drowning.
    D. Depth asphyxia.

Answers to Questions from page 24

131. (D) COPD is a progressive disease. Degenerative alveolar changes and uneven distribution of ventilation promote an increasing discrepancy between ventilation and perfusion.

132. (A) Incidence of COPD has been shown to correlate with chronic bronchial irritation, as in cigarette smoking and urban air pollution.

133. (C) Distant breath sounds are consistent with emphysema, especially in patients with increased AP chest diameter.

134. (C) Respiratory and heart rates are often rapid. Degenerative alveolar changes increase dead space ventilation, increasing the work of breathing.

135. (C) Decreased tissue oxygen supply causes the body to attempt to compensate by manufacturing more erythrocytes, resulting in polycythemia. Bullae result from loss of elastic tissue in the affected area.

136. (B) Polycythemia causes increased viscosity of blood, resulting in increased risk for pulmonary emboli.

149. The pathophysiology of acute pulmonary inhalation injuries due to thermal injury to lung tissues leads to mucosal sloughing, bronchorrhea, and

    A. Decreased mucus production.
    B. No significant change in ventilation-perfusion.
    C. Bradypnea.
    D. Pulmonary edema.

150. Which of the following statements regarding carbon monoxide (CO) toxicity is *false*?

    A. Carbon monoxide has an affinity for hemoglobin 200–250 times that of oxygen.
    B. Treatment consists of oxygenation with an initially low FI_{O_2}, which is slowly increased.
    C. Patients with CO toxicity may manifest personality changes and impaired judgment.
    D. A diagnostic indicator for CO poisoning is carboxyhemoglobin analysis.

Answers to Questions from page 25

137. **(A)** When an asthmatic patient is confronted with irritating stimuli, the bronchial tree becomes hyperreactive, resulting in bronchospasm. The narrowed airways compound the coexistent problem of excessive mucus production.

138. **(C)** In response to bronchial hyperreactivity, airway passages narrow and wheezing becomes apparent. As the bronchospasm and mucus production continue, the work of breathing increases, leading ultimately to a rapid respiratory rate and physical exhaustion. Dehydration may eventually result from continuous insensible water loss through the lungs.

139. **(A)** Owing to the increased insensible water loss through the lungs, asthmatic patients require administration of fluids and humidification.

140. **(A)** Chest pain is not always seen in pulmonary embolus. The most reliable symptoms are dyspnea and tachypnea.

141. **(C)** Characteristics of the pain seen with pulmonary embolus are: sudden in onset, laterally located, sharp in nature, and aggravated by respiration.

142. **(A)** Streptokinase facilitates the conversion of plasminogen to active plasmin. Plasmin dissolves fibrin, which is responsible for clot formation.

143. **(B)** In flail chest, chest wall instability results from the fracture of several adjacent ribs. The affected section moves opposite to that of the remaining chest wall, thus impairing ventilation.

Answers to Questions from page 26	Answers to Questions from page 27

144. **(A)** In tension pneumothorax, the pleura rises because air is entering the pleural space. This positive pressure compresses the lung on the affected side and causes the trachea to deviate toward the unaffected side.

145. **(C)** Aortic tear or rupture may result from injuries causing rapid deceleration. Symptoms may include a pulse difference in upper and lower extremities, blood pressure differences between the right and left arms, chest pain, and backache. A murmur may be heard anteriorly over the precordium and posteriorly between the scapulae.

146. **(D)** Protective laryngeal mechanisms are likely to be impaired after long-term intubation. These diminished responses predispose the patient to aspiration. Mercury-tipped enteral feeding tubes are positioned in the duodenum.

147. **(C)** Alveolar surfactant may be affected in aspiration of either fresh or salt water. Fresh water removes or displaces surfactant more significantly than salt water.

148. **(B)** Fresh water is hypotonic to body fluid; therefore, it diffuses out of the alveoli rapidly into the vascular space.

149. **(D)** Irritation to respiratory tissues in thermal injuries leads to pulmonary edema. Patients with such injuries also produce copious amounts of mucus, have ventilation-perfusion inequalities, and will be tachypneic.

150. **(B)** Carbon monoxide–toxic patients require immediate oxygenation at a high (100%) $F_{I_{O_2}}$. If hyperbaric oxygenation apparatus is available, its use would be appropriate.

Bibliography

American Association of Critical-Care Nurses: Core Curriculum for Critical Care Nursing, 3rd ed. W. B. Saunders Co., Philadelphia, 1985.
Text is presented in a systems approach, utilizing outline format. Includes salient points relevant to each system. Good text for delineating essential information for critical care nursing. Appropriate for practitioners, educators, and students.

Bates, B.: A Guide to Physical Examination, 3rd ed. J. B. Lippincott Co., Philadelphia, 1983.
Provides a good description of normal physical findings. Presents physical assessment techniques in a basic, easily understood manner. Contains numerous helpful illustrations.

Budassi, S. A., and Barber, J. M.: Emergency Nursing Principles and Practice. C. V. Mosby Co., St. Louis, 1981.
Deals thoroughly with acute interventions appropriate in all types of emergency situations. Includes brief discussion of pathophysiology. Numerous illustrations enhance content. Excellent comprehensive appendices, such as legal standards, pharmacology, and laboratory values.

Ganong, W. F.: Review of Medical Physiology, 11th ed. Lange Medical Publications, Inc., Los Altos, 1983.
A concise advanced human physiology test that also includes brief reviews of related anatomy throughout. Contains limited symptomatology of some physiological disorders.

Harper, R. W.: A Guide to Respiratory Care: Physiological and Clinical Applications. J. B. Lippincott Co., Philadelphia, 1981.
Respiratory text written for nurses that provides a thorough discussion of physiology. Illustrations and tables greatly enhance the content. Study questions are included at the end of each chapter. Contains very useful appendices.

Hudak, C. M., Lohr, T., and Gallo, B. M. (eds.): Critical Care Nursing, 3rd ed. J. B. Lippincott Co., Philadelphia, 1982.
A critical care text that summarizes essential information for understanding conditions requiring acute interventions. Easy to read and understand.

Johanson, B. C., Dungca, C. U., Hoffmeister, D. and Wells, S. J. (eds.): Standards for Critical Care. C. V. Mosby Co., St. Louis, 1981.
Topics are presented in nursing process format, beginning with brief pathophysiologic discussion of the disease process. Relevant assessment data is identified. Potential problems and their symptoms are enumerated for each topic. Goals of care and a comprehensive outline of nursing activities are provided.

Kinney, M. R., Dear, C. B., Packa, D. R., and Voorman, D. M. (eds.): AACN's Clinical Reference for Critical Care Nursing. McGraw-Hill Book Co., New York, 1981.
A very comprehensive text for critical care nurses. Separate chapters deal with physiology and pathophysiology of body systems.

Larson, E. L. and Vazquez, M. (eds.): Critical Care Nursing. W. B. Saunders Co., Philadelphia, 1983.
An excellent quick reference for critical care nurses. Addresses wide variety of clinical disorders, including an overview of the disorder, pertinent assessment, and priorities of nursing management. Excellent appendices for quick reference.

McIntyre, K. M., and Lewis, A. J. (eds.): Textbook of Advanced Cardiac Life Support. American Heart Association, Dallas, 1981.
Concisely summarizes critical concepts of advanced life support. Information is all current and documented throughout with recent research findings.

Petersdorf, R. G., Adams, R. D., Braunwald, E., Isselbacher, K. J., and Wilson, J. D. (eds.): Harrison's Principles of Internal Medicine, 10th ed. McGraw-Hill Book Co., New York, 1983.
An excellent resource containing exhaustive content relevant to internal medicine. Provides a good understanding of pathophysiological basis for diseases as well as appropriate treatment.

Shapiro, B. A., Harrison, R. A., and Trout, C. A.: Clinical Application of Respiratory Care, 2nd ed. Year Book Medical Publishers, Inc., Chicago, 1979.
Comprehensive text dealing with clinical respiratory care. Gives both theoretical and clinical rationales for therapy. Pertinent points are summarized at the end of each chapter.

2 □ THE CARDIOVASCULAR SYSTEM

TERESA THOMA KEVIL
SUSAN ARMSTRONG SCREWS

1. Cardiac muscle can function as a syncytium because of the

   A. Abundance of ATP.
   B. Presence of intercalated disks.
   C. Presence of protoplasmic bridges.
   D. Absence of cell membranes.

2. Atrial contraction forces what portion of cardiac output into the ventricle?

   A. 100%.
   B. 70%.
   C. 30%.
   D. 15%.

3. The first heart sound, S_1, is related to which event in the cardiac cycle?

   A. Opening of atrioventricular valves.
   B. Closure of atrioventricular valves.
   C. Opening of semilunar valves.
   D. Closure of semilunar valves.

4. The heart sound that immediately precedes the carotid upstroke is

   A. S_1.
   B. S_2.
   C. S_3.
   D. S_4.

5. The second heart sound, S_2, is associated with which cardiac event?

   A. Opening of atrioventricular valves.
   B. Closure of atrioventricular valves.
   C. Opening of semilunar valves.
   D. Closure of semilunar valves.

6. The second heart sound is heard at the beginning of which phase of the cardiac cycle?

   A. Isovolumetric contraction.
   B. Atrial systole.
   C. Ventricular diastole.
   D. Ventricular systole.

7. The interval between the first and second heart sounds is ventricular

   A. Diastole.
   B. Systole.
   C. Presystole.
   D. Protodiastole.

8. In most cases, ischemia of the AV junction results from occlusion of which coronary artery?

   A. Left anterior descending.
   B. Left circumflex.
   C. Diagonal.
   D. Right.

9. Angiotensin II is a potent

   A. Vasodilator.
   B. Vasoconstrictor.
   C. Diuretic.
   D. Antihistamine.

10. A patient's blood pressure is 170/100. Her mean arterial pressure is

    A. 70 mm Hg.
    B. 93 mm Hg.
    C. 123 mm Hg.
    D. 203 mm Hg.

11. The effects of beta-adrenergic blocking agents include

    A. Increased heart rate.
    B. Enhanced myocardial contractility.
    C. Stimulation of renin secretion.
    D. Decreased myocardial oxygen consumption.

12. In sinus arrhythmia, intermittent slowing of the heart rate is correlated with which phase of ventilation?

   A. Between inspiration and expiration.
   B. Expiration.
   C. Early inspiration.
   D. Late inspiration.

13. The ability of the sinoatrial (SA) node to initiate an electrical impulse spontaneously is known as

   A. Automaticity.
   B. Rhythmicity.
   C. Contractility.
   D. Conductivity.

14. The brief impulse delay that occurs in the AV node allows time for

   A. Atrial depolarization.
   B. Atrial repolarization.
   C. Completion of atrial contraction.
   D. Completion of ventricular contraction.

15. The pressure in the left ventricle initially exceeds that in the aorta during

   A. Isovolumetric contraction.
   B. Ventricular ejection.
   C. Isovolumetric relaxation.
   D. Ventricular filling.

16. The tension of the ventricle immediately preceding systole is referred to as

   A. Preload.
   B. Afterload.
   C. Pulmonary vascular resistance.
   D. Systemic vascular resistance.

17. The force that the left ventricle must generate to eject its blood volume is referred to as

   A. Pulmonary vascular resistance.
   B. Afterload.
   C. Preload.
   D. Cardiac index.

Answers to Questions from page 31

1. (**B**) Cardiac muscle may depolarize in a "rippling" manner because of the presence of low-resistance connections created by intercalated discs.

2. (**C**) During diastole, the ventricle fills approximately 70% passively. Atrial contraction provides an additional 30%, completing ventricular filling. This 30% is known as the "atrial kick."

3. (**B**) S_1 is attributed to vibrations set up by closure of the atrioventricular valves. There are two major components of S_1, M_1 (mitral valve closure) and T_1 (tricuspid valve closure).

4. (**A**) S_1 is heard immediately preceding the carotid upstroke and occurs approximately simultaneously with the apical impulse.

5. (**D**) The second heart sound results from vibrations set up by the closure of the aortic and pulmonic valves. Two components of S_2 are A_2 (aortic valve closure) and P_2 (pulmonic valve closure).

6. (**C**) S_2, associated with closure of the semilunar valves, occurs at the onset of ventricular diastole.

18. For a patient with a thermodilution catheter and arterial line in place, readings for the past hour were as follows:

Mean right atrial pressure	16 mm Hg
Mean pulmonary artery pressure	20 mm Hg
Cardiac output	5.2 L/min.
Systolic BP	140 mm Hg
Diastolic BP	90 mm Hg
Mean arterial BP	106 mm Hg

This patient's systemic vascular resistance (SVR) is:

A. 1138 dynes/sec/cm^2.
B. 1323 dynes/sec/cm^2.
C. 1384 dynes/sec/cm^2.
D. 1730 dynes/sec/cm^2.

19. Factors that increase myocardial contractility include

A. Hyperkalemia.
B. Beta-adrenergic blockade.
C. Parasympathetic stimulation.
D. Sympathetic stimulation.

20. The component of a health history that briefly describes the patient's presenting problem in his own words is the

A. History of present illness.
B. Chief complaint.
C. Past medical history.
D. Social history.

21. The most reliable vessel to utilize when estimating central venous pressure (CVP) is the

A. External jugular vein.
B. Subclavian vein.
C. Saphenous vein.
D. Internal jugular vein.

22. A physical assessment finding indicative of right heart failure is

A. The presence of hepatojugular reflux.
B. The presence of Homan's sign.
C. The presence of the oculocephalic reflex.
D. A positive Allen test.

Answers to Questions from page 32

7. (**B**) S_1 marks the onset of systole and S_2 the onset of diastole. Therefore, the time between S_1 and S_2 is systole, whereas the time between S_2 and the next S_1 is diastole.

8. (**D**) In most (90%) people, the AV node is supplied by the right coronary artery. For the remainder of the population it is supplied by the circumflex branch of the left coronary artery.

9. (**B**) Angiotensin II is one of the most potent vasoconstrictors known. Hypotension stimulates the release of renin, which converts angiotensin I to angiotensin II. In addition to potent vasoconstriction, angiotensin II stimulates release of aldosterone from the adrenal cortex.

10. (**C**) Mean arterial pressure (MAP) may be estimated by adding the diastolic blood pressure and one-third of the pulse pressure. With the values given, the MAP is:

$$100 + \tfrac{1}{3}(70) = 100 + 23 = 123$$

Another formula for estimating MAP is

$$\frac{\text{Systolic Blood Pressure} + 2(\text{Diastolic Blood Pressure})}{3}$$

With the values given, the calculation is:

$$\frac{170 + 2(100)}{3} = \frac{370}{3} = 123$$

Normal parameters for MAP are 70–110 mm Hg.

11. (**D**) Beta-adrenergic blocking agents, such as propranolol, decrease heart rate and myocardial contractility, thus decreasing myocardial oxygen consumption.

23. The abnormality present when there is a greater than 10 mm Hg drop in arterial systolic pressure on inspiration is called pulsus

    A. Alternans.
    B. Magnus.
    C. Paradoxus.
    D. Parvus.

24. When palpating the precordium of an adult patient, the nurse would expect to find the apical impulse in the

    A. Left 4th intercostal space lateral to the midclavicular line.
    B. Right 2nd intercostal space at the right sternal border.
    C. Left 5th intercostal space at the midclavicular line.
    D. Left 5th intercostal space at the midaxillary line.

25. The first heart sound (S_1) is produced by

    A. Closure of the mitral and tricuspid valves.
    B. Ventricular filling.
    C. Closure of the aortic and pulmonic valves.
    D. Atrial filling.

26. Which of the following statements is true regarding the second heart sound (S_2)?

    A. It is produced by closure of the mitral and aortic valves.
    B. It occurs at the end of ventricular diastole.
    C. It is heard loudest at the apex.
    D. Its component parts can be heard more distinctly on inspiration.

27. When auscultating the precordium of a 64-year-old male patient, you detect a third heart sound (S_3). Your interpretation is that an S_3 is

    A. Normally heard in elderly individuals.
    B. Always a pathological finding.
    C. A high-pitched sound heard best with the diaphragm.
    D. Due to resistance to ventricular filling.

Answers to Questions from page 33

12. (**B**) In sinus arrhythmia of respiratory origin, decrease in heart rate occurs with expiration. Heart rate increases with inspiration. This mecanism is called the *respiratory reflex* and is caused by inhibition of vagal tone. The augmentation of venous return that results is sometimes referred to as the *respiratory pump*.

13. (**A**) Automaticity, the ability to generate an electrical impulse spontaneously, is a property of the SA node. The AV junction, bundle branches, and peripheral Purkinje fibers also contain pacemaker cells that possess this property. The SA node normally serves as the "pacemaker," because its rate of automaticity is faster than that of other pacemaker cells.

14. (**C**) The P wave on the ECG denotes atrial depolarization. Atrial contraction occurs immediately after depolarization. The brief (about 0.10 second) delay of the impulse that occurs in the AV node is inscribed on the ECG as the isoelectric portion of the P-R interval (P-R segment). During this time, the atria contract and complete ventricular filling.

15. (**A**) Ventricular systole begins with isovolumetric contraction. As the ventricles contract, the AV valves close, and the left ventricular pressure rises until it exceeds that in the aorta and pulmonary artery. When this occurs, the semilunar valves open and the ejection phase of ventricular systole begins.

16. (**A**) Preload is related to the stretch, or tension and volume, of the ventricle at the end of diastole. The concept of preload is based on the Frank-Starling law: Within physiologic limits, the ventricle will alter contractile force to pump the volume of blood that enters it. Demands beyond physiologic limits result in heart failure.

17. (**B**) The resistance that the left ventricle must overcome to empty is referred to as *afterload*. It can be estimated indirectly through calculation of systemic vascular resistance.

28. A fourth heart sound (S_4) is also called a(n) _____ gallop.

    A. Atrial.
    B. Summation.
    C. Ventricular.
    D. Systolic.

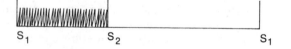

S_1 S_2 S_1

29. The murmur diagrammed above is a(n) _____ murmur.

    A. Protodiastolic.
    B. Pansystolic.
    C. Systolic ejection.
    D. Presystolic.

30. Your patient has a grade IV/VI systolic ejection murmur. This means that the murmur

    A. Is barely audible.
    B. Can be heard with the stethoscope off the chest.
    C. Can be heard well and is usually associated with a thrill.
    D. Is just easily audible.

31. Which of the following valvular defects results in a pansystolic murmur?

    A. Mitral stenosis.
    B. Aortic stenosis.
    C. Mitral insufficiency.
    D. Aortic insufficiency.

32. Which of the following congenital heart defects results in a pansystolic murmur?

    A. Interventricular septal defect.
    B. Coarctation of the aorta.
    C. Pulmonary stenosis.
    D. Patent ductus arteriosus.

Answers to Questions from page 34

18. **(C)** $$\text{SVR} = \frac{\text{Mean Arterial Pressure} - \text{Right Atrial Pressure (CVP)}}{\text{Cardiac Output}} \times 80$$

    SVR is analogous to afterload. Normal parameters vary with different authorities from 800–1500 dynes/sec/cm^2.

19. **(D)** Sympathetic stimulation increases contractility of the myocardium in part through the action of norepinephrine. Norepinephrine acts on beta-adrenergic receptors to increase heart rate and enhance myocardial contractility.

20. **(B)** The chief complaint is a very brief statement of the reason the patient is seeking medical care. The history of present illness is a detailed evaluation of the chief complaint. The past medical history explores previous illnesses, operations, and injuries. The social history contains a profile of the patient's activities of daily living, environment, habits, and interpersonal relationships.

21. **(D)** The internal jugular veins are the most reliable for estimating CVP. Information obtained by measuring these vessels relates to pressure and volume changes in the right atrium. The external jugular veins are less optimal for estimating central venous pressure because of the presence of venous valves between the superior vena cava and the external jugular veins. The subclavian veins are not used to estimate CVP, nor are the saphenous veins, which are located in the legs.

22. **(A)** The presence of hepatojugular reflux (HJR) is indicative of right heart failure. The technique for eliciting it consists of compressing for 30 to 45 seconds the upper abdomen of a patient elevated to 45 degree. The presence of HJR is indicated by an increase in the height of the distended jugular veins. Homan's sign is indicative of thrombophlebitis of the calf. Looking for the oculocephalic reflex, also called doll's eye movements, helps determine whether the brain stem is intact. The Allen test checks patency of ulnar arteries and collateral arteries of the hand.

33. Which of the following diagnostic procedures is most useful in determining cardiac ejection fraction?

    A. Thallium-201 scan.
    B. Technetium pyrophosphate imaging.
    C. Multiple gated acquisition scan.
    D. Echocardiography.

34. A normal ejection fraction obtained by MUGA scan would be a value of

    A. 35%.
    B. 50%.
    C. 65%.
    D. 100%.

35. Which of the following statements regarding the electrocardiogram (ECG) is *true*?

    A. It measures electrical activity of the heart.
    B. It cannot provide information about the size of the heart chambers.
    C. It documents muscular contraction of the heart.
    D. It cannot indicate electrolyte imbalances.

36. The characteristic of ECG recording paper that allows us to measure a P-R interval is

    A. The horizontal lines.
    B. The vertical lines.
    C. The 3-second markers.
    D. None of above.

37. When an electrical impulse moves *away* from a positive electrode, what type of deflection is seen on the ECG?

    A. Positive
    B. Diphasic.
    C. Isoelectric.
    D. Negative.

Answers to Questions from page 35

23. **(C)** During inspiration, there is a normal drop in arterial systolic pressure. *A drop in pressure exceeding 10 mm Hg* is called pulsus paradoxus. This abnormality occurs with obstruction to venous return, which can be found in constrictive pericardial disease and severe obstructive pulmonary disease. *Pulsus alternans* refers to a variation in amplitude of the pulse from beat to beat. *Pulsus magnus* is a strong, bounding pulse. *Pulsus parvus* is a small, weak pulse.

24. **(C)** In adults, the apical impulse is normally found in the left 5th intercostal space at the midclavicular line. In children the apical impulse can be found in the left 4th intercostal space until age 7. It is lateral to the midclavicular line until age 4. The right 2nd intercostal space at the right sternal border is the aortic area. Lateral displacement of the apical impulse toward the axilla may indicate several things, including left ventricular hypertrophy.

25. **(A)** Closure of the mitral and tricuspid valves produces the first heart sound. Because the ventricles contract asynchronously, mitral valve closure slightly precedes tricuspid valve closure. However, S_1 is normally heard as a single sound. It signifies the beginning of ventricular systole and is loudest at the apex.

26. **(D)** S_2 is produced by the closure of the aortic and pulmonic valves. Aortic valve closure precedes pulmonic valve closure. This physiologic occurrence—differing closure times—becomes more pronounced on inspiration, when pulmonic valve closure is further delayed. S_2 occurs at the end of ventricular systole and is loudest at the base of the heart.

27. **(D)** S_3 occurs because of resistance to ventricular filling. Its presence can be either physiologic or pathologic. A physiologic S_3 is common in children and young adults. An S_3 is a low-pitched sound heard best with the bell of the stethoscope.

38. The ECG waveform indicative of atrial depolarization is the _____wave.

    A. Q.
    B. P.
    C. T.
    D. U.

39. The P-R interval is significant because it

    A. Measures conduction velocity through the ventricles.
    B. Measures total ventricular depolarization.
    C. Represents atrial depolarization and conduction through the AV node.
    D. Represents ventricular depolarization and repolarization, or electrical systole.

40. Which of the following measurements would be considered normal for a P-R interval?

    A. 0.06 seconds.
    B. 0.16 seconds.
    C. 0.24 seconds.
    D. 0.32 seconds.

41. Ventricular hypertrophy can be diagnosed on an ECG by several features, including

    A. Increased R wave amplitude.
    B. Abnormal heart rate.
    C. Tall, peaked T waves.
    D. Wide, notched P waves.

42. You evaluate a monitor strip and find that the patient's QRS interval is 0.14 seconds. You are aware that this is

    A. Normal.
    B. At the upper limits of normal, so the patient requires observation.
    C. Abnormal but insignificant.
    D. Abnormal and indicative of impaired ventricular conduction.

Answers to Questions from page 36

28. (A) An S_4 is called an atrial or presystolic gallop. It is due to overloading of either ventricle and/or increased diastolic pressure. An S_3 is called a ventricular gallop. A summation gallop is the single sound produced by the merging of both an S_3 and an S_4 in rapid heart rates.

29. (B) The murmur diagrammed is a pansystolic or holosystolic murmur. It is heard throughout systole. A protodiastolic murmur is heard in early diastole. A systolic ejection murmur starts after S_1 and ends before S_2. A presystolic murmur is heard in late diastole.

30. (C) A grade IV/VI murmur is one that can be heard well and is usually associated with a thrill. A grade I/VI murmur is barely audible. A grade II/VI murmur is just easily audible. A grade III/VI murmur can be heard well. A grade V/VI murmur is loud but requires a stethoscope. A grade VI/VI murmur is very loud and can be heard with the stethoscope off the chest.

31. (C) Mitral insufficiency or regurgitation results in a pansystolic murmur. Because the incompetent valve cannot effectively close during ventricular systole, blood not only exits through the aortic valve into the aorta but also regurgitates back into the left atrium through the incompetent valve. Mitral stenosis results in a mid-diastolic and/or presystolic murmur. Aortic stenosis results in a systolic ejection murmur. Aortic insufficiency results in a pandiastolic murmur.

32. (A) Interventricular septal defects result in pansystolic murmurs. Coarctation of the aorta results in a systolic ejection murmur. Pulmonary stenosis results in a loud systolic ejection murmur. Patent ductus arteriosus results in a continuous murmur, involving systole and diastole.

43. In patients with acute transmural myocardial infarction, the S-T segment is characteristically

    A. Isoelectric.
    B. Elevated.
    C. Prolonged.
    D. Depressed.

44. An example of a unipolar precordial lead is

    A. II.
    B. aVR.
    C. aVF.
    D. V_1.

45. Which of the following statements about lead MCL_1 is *false*?

    A. It allows for differentiation between aberrancy and ventricular ectopy.
    B. The QRS complex is primarily a positive deflection.
    C. It allows for differentiation between right and left ventricular ectopy.
    D. It allows for early detection of dysrhythmias and ischemia.

46. The salient feature of a sinus arrhythmia is that the

    A. Rhythm and rate vary with the ventilatory cycle.
    B. Rate is below 60 per minute.
    C. QRS duration varies with the ventilatory cycle.
    D. Morphology of the P waves varies significantly.

47. Which of the following dysrhythmias should the nurse *not* expect to see in patients with sick sinus syndrome?

    A. Sinus bradycardia.
    B. Sinus exit block.
    C. Complete heart block.
    D. Supraventricular tachyarrhythmias.

Answers to Questions from page 37

33. (**C**) The multiple gated acquisition (MUGA) scan involves tagging RBCs with technetium and obtaining images of cardiac volumes in systole and diastole. The analysis of these data provides a measurement of the ejection fraction (EF), one of the indices of ventricular function. Thallium-210 is used in myocardial perfusion imaging for identification of ischemic areas. Technetium pyrophosphate is used for myocardial infarct imaging. Echocardiography is useful for differential diagnosis in mitral valve disease and pericardial effusion.

34. (**C**) A normal ejection fraction is 65%, plus or minus 10%. Lower ejection fraction values are indicative of ventricular dysfunction.

35. (**A**) The ECG measures electrical activity of the heart. It can indicate anatomical alterations, chamber hypertrophy, electrolyte imbalances, and toxicity of certain drugs. The ECG does not document mechanical activity of the heart.

36. (**B**) The vertical lines on ECG paper measure time. Small (1-mm) boxes equal 0.04 seconds each and large (5-mm) boxes equal 0.20 seconds each. These lines allow us to measure time periods such as the P-R interval. The horizontal lines on ECG paper measure voltage. The 3-second markers are displayed above the graph portion of the paper and are used to calculate heart rates.

37. (**D**). When an electrical impulse moves away from a positive electrode, it produces a negative deflection. A positive deflection occurs when an electrical impulse moves toward a positive electrode. Diphasic deflections occur when an electrical impulse moves both toward and away from (i.e., perpendicular or at 90° to) a positive electrode. The isoelectric line indicates either that there are no electrical forces or that there are equal amounts of movement toward and away from a positive electrode.

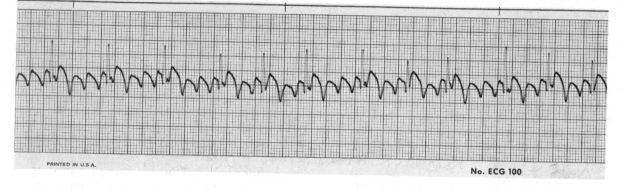

PRINTED IN U.S.A.   No. ECG 100

48. The rhythm displayed on the above ECG strip is

    A. Ventricular flutter.
    B. Mobitz II block.
    C. Atrial flutter.
    D. Atrial fibrillation.

49. Premature ventricular contractions (PVCs) warrant immediate attention if:

    A. R on T phenomenon is present.
    B. They assume left bundle configuration.
    C. No pulse is felt with premature beat.
    D. The patient senses the "skipped beats."

50. A dysrhythmia characterized by erratic undulating waveforms in place of identifiable QRS complexes is

    A. Atrial flutter.
    B. Junctional tachycardia.
    C. Ventricular tachycardia.
    D. Ventricular fibrillation.

51. A *true* statement concerning conduction in first-degree AV block is that

    A. The impulse arises from the AV junction.
    B. Conduction is abnormally slowed across the AV junction.
    C. It results from failure of the SA node.
    D. The P wave is unusually wide.

52. An arrhythmia characterized by cycles in which the P-R interval progressively lengthens until a QRS complex is dropped is called

    A. Sinus arrest.
    B. Wenckebach phenomenon.
    C. Mobitz II second-degree AV block.
    D. Third-degree heart block.

Answers to Questions from page 38

38. (**B**) The P wave indicates atrial depolarization. The Q wave marks the onset of ventricular depolarization. The T wave represents ventricular repolarization. The U wave is thought to be significant in hypokalemic states.

39. (**C**) The P-R interval represents atrial depolarization and includes the normal delay of the impulse of the AV node. The QRS complex measures total ventricular depolarization. The Q-T interval represents ventricular depolarization and repolarization, or electrical systole.

40. (**B**) A normal P-R interval falls between 0.12 and 0.20 seconds. A shortened P-R interval would indicate accelerated conduction. A lengthened P-R interval would indicate delayed conduction, such as occurs with first-degree heart block.

41. (**A**) Ventricular hypertrophy can be diagnosed on ECG by several factors, including increased amplitude of the R wave in selected V leads. Wide, notched P waves may indicate atrial hypertrophy.

42. (**D**) A normal QRS interval is 0.06 to 0.10 seconds. This measurement indicates the time involved in total ventricular depolarization. An interval greater than 0.12 seconds indicates delayed conduction, such as that seen in bundle branch block.

53. Complete heart block (CHB) or third-degree heart block is characterized by

    A. A ventricular rate faster than the atrial rate.
    B. P waves occasionally conducted to ventricles.
    C. A total loss of conduction through the AV junction.
    D. An irregular ventricular rhythm.

54. One characteristic of right bundle branch block is

    A. Abnormal left ventricular depolarization.
    B. Septum depolarizing from the left.
    C. An rSR′ in left lateral precordial leads.
    D. Delayed depolarization of RV.

55. Tall, peaked T waves are characteristic of which electrolyte disturbance?

    A. Hyperkalemia.
    B. Hypokalemia.
    C. Hypercalcemia.
    D. Hyponatremia.

56. Which of the following suggests quinidine toxicity?

    A. Widening of QRS complex.
    B. Diarrhea.
    C. Tinnitus.
    D. Skin rash.

57. Beta-adrenergic blocking agents constitute which group of antiarrhythmics?

    A. Group II.
    B. Group III.
    C. Group IV.
    D. Group V.

Answers to Questions from page 39

43. (**B**) The ECG of transmural myocardial infarction patients characteristically shows S-T elevation. This segment may also be elevated with pericarditis or aneurysm. A depressed S-T segment may indicate angina, right ventricular hypertrophy, or digitalis toxicity and may be seen in patients with subendocardial myocardial infarction. A prolonged S-T segment is indicative of hypocalcemia. Normally the S-T segment is isoelectric.

44. (**D**) The six V leads are unipolar precordial or chest leads. Leads I, II, and III are bipolar limb leads. The augmented unipolar limb leads include aVR, aVL, and aVF.

45. (**B**) In a modified chest lead (MCL₁), the QRS pattern is typically negative.

46. (**A**) In sinus arrhythmia, the rhythm and rate vary with the ventilatory cycle. This variety is thought to be due to circulatory reflexes that occur with changes in intrathoracic pressure, resulting in irregular P-P (and R-R) intervals. The rate is faster on inspiration and slower on expiration. The QRS interval remains constant, as does the P wave morphology.

47. (**C**) Sick sinus syndrome is thought to be related to degeneration of cells in the SA node. The syndrome is characterized by a combination of sinus bradycardia, supraventricular tachyarrhythmias, and sinus exit block.

58. Pharmacologic actions most effective in suppressing ventricular tachycardia and fibrillation are associated with which group of antiarrhythmic agents?

   A. Group III.
   B. Group IV.
   C. Group V.
   D. Group VI.

59. Group V antiarrhythmic agents act by

   A. Calcium ion antagonism.
   B. Decreasing membrane conductance.
   C. Beta-adrenergic receptor blockade.
   D. Making the RMP more negative.

60. A noninvasive method of detecting coronary artery disease (CAD) is

   A. Cardiac catheterization.
   B. Holter monitoring.
   C. Exercise stress test.
   D. MUGA scanning.

61. A test useful in documenting the effectiveness of antiarrhythmic therapy is

   A. Cardiac catheterization.
   B. Exercise electrocardiogram.
   C. Cardiac CAT scanning.
   D. Holter monitoring.

Answers to Questions from page 40

48. (C) The illustrated ECG strip demonstrates atrial flutter. The flutter waves have a characteristic sawtooth appearance. The conduction ratio may be constant or variable. The strip shows atrial flutter with varying degrees (4:1 and 3:1) of block.

49. (A) Premature ventricular contractions are potentially dangerous if they are more frequent than 6/minute, multiform or coupled or if they occur on the T wave of the preceding beat. Owing to the shortened filling time of the ventricle, which is due to the PVCs, a pulse is frequently absent. When R on T phenomenon is present, the premature beat occurs in the supernormal phase of the refractory period and could precipitate an episode of ventricular tachycardia or fibrillation.

50. (D) In ventricular fibrillation, there are no discernible complexes. The erratic baseline characteristic of ventricular fibrillation results from uncoordinated ventricular depolarization. Ventricular contractions do not occur, and death ensues if the dysrhythmia persists.

51. (B) In first-degree AV block, the impulse arises normally from the SA node so that a "normal" P wave is inscribed. Conduction from the atria to the ventricles, however, is delayed excessively through the AV junction. First-degree AV block is manifest by a P-R interval greater than .20 seconds in duration. The P-R interval is measured from the beginning of the P wave to the beginning of the QRS complex.

52. (B) The description above characterizes a second-degree heart block, Mobitz I or Wenckebach. It is due to the progressive slowing of conduction across the AV junction. The abnormality is usually in the AV node. In each complex, the P-R interval lengthens and the R-R interval shortens until a beat is dropped (nonconducted P wave), resulting in the appearance of group beating.

62. A male patient ejects 50 ml from his left ventricle with each heart beat. His heart rate is 120. What is his cardiac output (C.O.)?

    A. 2.4 L/min.
    B. 3 L/min.
    C. 5 L/min.
    D. 6 L/min.

63. Your patient is 5'4" tall, weighs 125 pounds, and her cardiac output is 6 L/min. What is her cardiac index (CI)?

    A. 2.8.
    B. 3.8.
    C. 4.0.
    D. 4.4.

64. A diagnostic test used to confirm coronary artery disease is

    A. Echocardiogram.
    B. Electrocardiogram.
    C. Cardiac catheterization.
    D. Ventriculogram.

Answers to Questions from page 41

53. (**C**) In the third-degree heart block, the atria and ventricles beat independently of one another. There is no consistent relationship between P waves and QRS complexes. P waves are not conducted to the ventricles. Ventricular beats may arise from the AV junction or the ventricles. Ventricular rates vary on the basis of the location of the pacemaker, but rates are generally slow and regular.

54. (**D**) When conduction in one of the bundle branches is interrupted, the impulse travels normally down the unaffected bundle. The wave of depolarization spreads to the ventricle served by the blocked bundles, resulting in delayed activation of that ventricle. The QRS complex is therefore widened to more than .10 seconds in duration. In right bundle branch block, the septum and left ventricle are depolarized normally, and the wave of depolarization spreads from left to right. An rSR' is inscribed in the *right* precordial leads (V_1 and V_2).

55. (**A**) Electrolyte abnormalities may cause a variety of electrocardiographic changes. Hyperkalemia is associated with tall, narrow, "pointed" T waves, P waves of diminished voltage, AV and intraventricular conduction delays, and increased QRS duration. Loss of P wave and widening of QRS are associated with severe hyperkalemia (i.e., 8.5 mEq/L). Electrocardiographic changes seen in hyperkalemia disappear with resolution of hyperkalemia.

56. (**A**) Quinidine, a group I antiarrhythmic agent, slows conduction through the ventricles. Quinidine toxicity may result in an exaggeration of this effect, producing widened QRS, prolonged Q-T interval, heart block, or asystole. Gastrointestinal disturbances are the most common side effects. Side effects do not denote toxicity.

57. (**B**) Beta-adrenergic blocking agents form antiarrhythmic group III. The most commonly used drug of this group is propranolol.

65. Which would be *least* helpful detecting poor ventricular wall motion?

    A. Electrocardiogram.
    B. Echocardiogram.
    C. Radionuclide scanning (e.g., MUGA).
    D. Ventriculogram.

66. Motion picture filming during invasive procedures is known as

    A. Arteriography.
    B. Cineangiography.
    C. MUGA scanning.
    D. Fluoroscopy.

67. For coronary angiography, the catheter would probably be inserted via the

    A. Brachial artery.
    B. Femoral vein.
    C. Carotid artery.
    D. Subclavian vein.

68. Symptoms of cardiac tamponade include

    A. Increased cardiac output.
    B. Diminished atrial pressures.
    C. Paradoxical pulse.
    D. Intensified heart sounds.

69. If a pulmonary artery catheter is thought to be unintentionally wedged, appropriate measures would include all of the following *except*

    A. Filling the balloon to manipulate the tip.
    B. Checking to assure the balloon is deflated.
    C. Instructing the patient to cough.
    D. Pulling back slightly on the catheter.

Answers to Questions from page 42

58. (**B**) Antiarrhythmic agent group IV increases the fibrillatory threshold of the ventricles. An example of a drug in this group is bretylium tosylate. It is recommended in advanced cardiac life support protocols for refractory ventricular tachycardia and ventricular fibrillation. Initial dosage is 5 mg/kg of body weight.

59. (**A**) Group V agents work by blocking slow calcium channels. In the heart, intracellular calcium affects excitation and conduction of cardiac muscle, regeneration and conduction of impulses in the AV node, automaticity of the SA and AV nodes, and contraction of smooth muscle in systemic and coronary vascular beds. Slowing the influx of calcium into the cell decreases automaticity of SA and AV nodes and prolongs AV nodal conduction. Verapamil is a major drug of this group. Rapid I.V. administration may result in bradycardia, hypotension, AV block, or asystole.

60. (**C**) Exercise electrocardiography is a noninvasive technique for detecting CAD. While heart rate, blood pressure and ECG are continuously monitored, the patient exercises according to one of many specific protocols. The ECG is observed for significant ST segment displacement. Exercise testing is safe when preceded by a careful cardiovascular examination and performed under carefully monitored conditions by a qualified practitioner.

61. (**D**) A 24-hour electrocardiogram may be used to evaluate the effectiveness of antiarrhythmic therapy. Frequency of arrhythmias may be correlated with peak and trough drug levels.

70. Ectopy from insertion of a thermodilution catheter would most likely occur while the catheter is passing through the

    A. Right atrium.
    B. Right ventricle.
    C. Left atrium.
    D. Left ventricle.

71. Which of the following would *not* be a major goal in planning care for the hospitalized cardiac patient?

    A. Maintain normal fluid and electrolyte balance.
    B. Maintain adequate nutrition.
    C. Keep free of infection.
    D. Encourage and schedule frequent activity.

72. Which of the following findings may indicate cardiovascular compromise in a patient with documented cardiac disease?

    A. Absence of a pulse deficit.
    B. Progressive mental confusion.
    C. A PCWP of 8 mm Hg.
    D. A serum potassium of 4.5 mEq/L.

73. Which of the following statements' regarding pulmonary artery catheters is *false*?

    A. Pressure readings can be obtained with the patient in semi-Fowler's position.
    B. Infection rarely occurs as a result of placement of this catheter.
    C. The balloon of the catheter should remain deflated while PCW pressures are not being obtained.
    D. The catheter can cause ventricular fibrillation.

74. In planning nutritional support for the cardiac patient, the nurse should realize that such a patient is most often put on a diet that is

    A. Sodium-free and cholesterol-free.
    B. Potassium-free.
    C. sodium-restricted and cholesterol-restricted.
    D. Potassium-restricted.

Answers to Questions from page 43

62. (**D**)

    Cardiac output

    $$= \text{Stroke Volume} \times \text{Heart Rate}$$
    $$= 50 \times 120$$
    $$= 6000 \text{ ml or 6 L/min}$$

    This calculation method can be used if stroke volume is known. A common bedside technique for calculation of cardiac output is the thermodilution method. With this technique, a specific volume of cold fluid is injected via a thermodilution catheter into the right atrium. A probe in the distal portion of the catheter then measures the temperature of blood in the pulmonary artery. The cardiac output is calculated using the degree of warming of the injectate. The longer the injectate stays in the right ventricle, the warmer the blood at the distal tip and the lower the cardiac output.

63. (**B**)

    $$\text{Cardiac Index} = \frac{\text{Cardiac Output}}{\text{Body Surface Area}}$$
    $$= \frac{6}{1.57}$$
    $$= 3.82$$

    Cardiac index incorporates the size of the patient and the cardiac output to provide a value that suggests the adequacy of the output for meeting the body needs. Body surface area is calculated from height and weight and is read from a nomogram chart.

64. (**C**) Cardiac catheterization is used to confirm suspected coronary artery lesions. During the procedure, a contrast medium is injected, making the blood flow through the coronary circulation visible. Echocardiography and ventriculography provide information about cardiac chambers and some valvular lesions. Electrocardiograms provide information about cardiac electrical activity.

75. Which of the following evaluation outcomes would be questionable for a cardiac patient?

    A. The patient will not gain more than 4–5 lb per week.
    B. The patient will be free of dysrhythmias.
    C. Invasive line sites will be free from infection.
    D. The patient will be alert and oriented.

76. Progressive occlusion of coronary arteries may be due to all the following *except*

    A. The deposit of fatty material beneath the vessel's intimal layer.
    B. The presence of collateral circulation.
    C. Platelet aggregation on an atheroma.
    D. Fibrosis of the vessel lining.

77. Which of the following people is *least* likely to develop coronary artery disease?

    A. A 65-year-old male executive who smokes.
    B. A 25-year-old housewife with diabetes mellitus.
    C. A 40-year-old male with hypertension.
    D. A 30-year-old female schoolteacher with premenstrual syndrome.

78. Percutaneous transluminal coronary angioplasty (PTCA) is a therapeutic technique most appropriate for patients who

    A. Have multiple-vessel coronary artery disease.
    B. Have disease of the distal coronary vessels.
    C. Have single-vessel, proximal disease.
    D. Are not candidates for coronary bypass surgery.

Answers to Questions from page 44

65. (**A**) Ventricular wall motion may be evaluated with noninvasive echocardiography or invasive radionuclide scanning via a contrast ventriculogram. Electrocardiography evaluates electrical activity.

66. (**B**) Cineangiography is the recording of moving films during radiopaque contrast imaging of the heart. The films allow for post-procedure review to validate findings.

67. (**A**) For study of the coronary arteries, the catheter is inserted via a peripheral artery to the aorta. After retrograde advancement, the tip is positioned into the coronary circulation, and contrast medium is hand-injected.

68. (**C**) Cardiac tamponade is the accumulation of blood in the pericardial sac, which results in impairment of pumping action of the heart. Symptoms include increased heart rate, narrowing pulse pressure (elevated venous pressure, low arterial pressure), faint heart sounds, elevated atrial pressures, and paradoxical pulse.

69. (**A**) When a thermodilution catheter becomes fixed in a wedge position, immediate attention is warranted. Potential causes include distal balloon migration and leaving the balloon inflated. First, assure that the balloon is deflated by opening the balloon lumen to air, allowing deflation. Next, have the patient cough. This may manipulate the catheter tip enough to relieve the "wedge." If these measures are unsuccessful, either notify M.D. or pull back slightly on catheter until the PA waveform appears, according to institution policy. If the catheter is thought to be wedged, filling the balloon could result in balloon rupture or complications of overwedging, such as pulmonary infarction and rupture. Catheter placement should be verified periodically with chest x-ray and constantly with waveform analysis. Remember that thermodilution injections may cause distal migration of the catheter by tightening the right ventricular loop.

79. Which of the following is *not* a likely complication during the immediate postoperative period in a patient who has had CABG surgery?

   A. Myocardial infarction.
   B. Respiratory failure.
   C. Post-pump psychosis.
   D. Liver failure.

80. One of the primary therapeutic actions of sodium nitroprusside is to

   A. Increase preload.
   B. Decrease afterload.
   C. Increase systemic vascular resistance.
   D. Decrease pulmonary vascular resistance.

81. The pharmacologic agent that increases renal and mesenteric blood flow at low dosage is

   A. Dopamine.
   B. Nitroglycerin.
   C. Dobutamine.
   D. Epinephrine.

82. Dobutamine stimulates beta$_1$-adrenergic receptors. Therefore, its site of action is

   A. Skeletal muscle.
   B. Smooth muscle.
   C. The heart.
   D. The lungs.

83. A patient receiving I.V. nitroglycerin is admitted to your unit. The infusion is mixed in a glass I.V. bottle and attached to regular I.V. tubing. It is being administered by infusion pump at a dose of 3 µg/kg/min. You should

   A. Remove the infusion pump because it destroys the medication.
   B. Reduce the dose to less than 1 µg/kg/min to avoid toxic effects.
   C. Replace the regular I.V. tubing with special nonabsorbing tubing.
   D. Stop the infusion immediately to determine the extent of the patient's symptoms.

Answers to Questions from page 45

70. (**B**) Ventricular ectopy most often occurs when the catheter passes through the right ventricle. The catheter does not pass through the left side of the heart. Should ectopy occur, prepare to administer lidocaine I.V. If ectopy is frequent, the catheter should be withdrawn slightly and not advanced again until the arrhythmia abates.

71. (**D**) The hospitalized cardiac patient requires both physical and psychological rest to reduce the workload on the heart. Because of extended periods of bedrest, it is also important to prevent complications of immobility.

72. (**B**) Owing to the brain's sensitivity to hypoxia, mental confusion may be a fairly early sign of decreased cerebrovascular perfusion. A pulse deficit, which is a difference between the apical and radial pulse rate, is an abnormal finding. The pulmonary capillary wedge pressure (PCWP) is normally 4–12 mm Hg. Normal serum potassium is generally in the range of 3.5–5.0 mEq/L.

73. (**B**) The most common complication of pulmonary artery catheters is infection. The insertion is a sterile procedure, and catheters generally should not be left in place longer than 72 hours. It is the nurse's responsibility to change I.V. tubings within the system and to perform sterile dressing changes on a routine basis. As long as the transducer is at the same level of phlebostatic axis, patients can be in any position for pressure readings.

74. (**C**) Cardiac patients are most often put on diets that are restricted in sodium and cholesterol. For the large number of cardiac patients on diuretics, it is not only essential to ensure adequate dietary intake of foods containing potassium, but also frequently necessary to give electrolyte supplements.

84. Which of the following statements regarding angina is *true*?

    A. It indicates that a small portion of myocardium has died and is malfunctional.
    B. It results from myocardial cells being temporarily deprived of oxygen.
    C. It always leads to a heart attack.
    D. It can be successfully cured by nitrates.

85. During a routine office visit, a 52-year-old woman tells her doctor that she has recently experienced three episodes of heavy chest pain that radiates down her left arm and to her left ear. The pain occurs while she is playing tennis and subsides with rest. Her ECG is normal. This description suggests that

    A. Her pain is probably of pulmonary origin.
    B. Her symptoms are most likely psychosomatic.
    C. She should be further evaluated for angina.
    D. She has had a myocardial infarction.

86. Which of the following ECG changes is suggestive of angina?

    A. Prolonged Q-T interval.
    B. Inverted P wave.
    C. Pronounced Q wave.
    D. S-T segment depression.

87. Which of the following drugs would be the *least* beneficial in terminating or eliminating an acute anginal attack?

    A. Digoxin.
    B. Propranolol.
    C. Nifedipine.
    D. Nitroglycerin.

88. The major thrust of nursing intervention for a patient with angina should be directed toward

    A. Patient and family education.
    B. Returning the patient to his or her previous lifestyle.
    C. Absolute, prolonged physical and emotional rest.
    D. Forcing the patient to accept that he or she can no longer lead a normal life.

Answers to Questions from page 46

75. (**A**) In establishing outcome criteria for the cardiac patient, the nurse should be aware that significant weight gain increases the workload of the heart as well as is a potential indicator of fluid overload. If weight gain is allowed, it should not exceed 1–2 lb per week. In those patients in congestive or edematous states, the nurse might establish criteria involving weight loss.

76. (**B**) The progressively occlusive atherosclerotic process in the coronary arteries compromises blood flow and oxygen delivery to the myocardium. Occlusion can occur as the result of fatty deposits beneath the vessel intima, platelet aggregation on an atheroma, and fibrosis of the vessel lining. As the occlusive process progresses, collateral circulation frequently develops to provide adequate perfusion of myocardial tissue.

77. (**D**) Several risk factors are associated with the development of coronary artery disease. These include heredity, hypertension, diabetes, aging, male sex, smoking, hyperlipidemia, obesity, stress, sedentary life style, and gout. The role of estrogen in premenopausal women is a protective one.

78. (**C**) PTCA is most appropriate for individuals who have single-vessel, proximal coronary artery disease. Patients should have good collateral circulation and be candidates for coronary artery bypass graft (CABG) surgery. PTCA is recommended in patients with noncalcified lesions; however, it has recently been utilized in patients with calcified lesions. The technique involves passing a balloon-tipped dilatation catheter into the affected vessel under fluoroscopic guidance. The balloon is then inflated to flatten the atheroma against the wall of the vessel, thus enlarging the vessel lumen.

89. Myocardial infarction (MI) differs from angina in that MI pain

    A. Occurs most often in the right side of the chest.
    B. Is not relieved by nitrates or rest.
    C. Has a shorter duration than anginal pain.
    D. Is the only symptom patients have.

90. In acute myocardial infarction, the cardiac enzyme that elevates most quickly and returns to normal the earliest is

    A. SGOT.
    B. LDH.
    C. CPK.
    D. SGPT.

91. A WBC count of 15,000 per mm³ 24 hours after admission for acute MI should be interpreted as

    A. Evidence that pneumonia has developed.
    B. A serious complication.
    C. Requiring immediate antibiotic therapy.
    D. A predictable response to myocardial injury.

92. Which of the following isoenzymes is cardiac-specific when elevated?

    A. LDH$_3$.
    B. CPK-MB.
    C. LDH$_5$.
    D. CPK-MM.

93. All of the following changes would be expected on the ECG of a recent MI patient, except

    A. An injury pattern.
    B. Ischemic changes.
    C. Evidence of hypertrophy.
    D. Evidence of necrosis.

Answers to Questions from page 47

79. (**D**) Complications that may occur immediately after CABG surgery include: low cardiac output syndrome, hemorrhage, hypertension, hypotension, cardiac tamponade, pericarditis, dysrhythmias, MI, respiratory failure, post-pump psychosis, and renal failure. Many of these complications result from extracorporeal circulation.

80. (**B**) One of the primary therapeutic actions of sodium nitroprusside is to decrease afterload. It does so by reducing total peripheral resistance. Because nitroprusside decreases left ventricular filling pressure, it also reduces preload.

81. (**A**) At low doses, dopamine HCL has a positive inotropic effect and also increases renal and mesenteric blood flow. Nitroglycerine directly dilates coronary arteries, thereby improving myocardial perfusion. It also causes some peripheral venous relaxation; however, at low doses, the direct cardiac effects are maintained without the systemic hemodynamic effects. Dobutamine has little direct effect on renal and mesenteric blood flow. Epinephrine increases systemic vascular resistance; this increase may compromise renal and mesenteric blood flow, even at lower dosages.

82. (**C**) Beta$_1$-adrenergic receptors are located in the heart. Stimulation results in increases in myocardial contractility, heart rate, and myocardial oxygen consumption. Beta$_2$ receptors are located in smooth muscle, and their stimulation results in vasodilatation. Stimulation of alpha receptors results in vasoconstriction.

83. (**C**) I.V. nitroglycerin absorbs into plastics, so it is mixed in glass bottles and hung with special nonabsorbant tubing. It must be administered by infusion pump for accuracy. Usual dosage is 1–4 μg/kg/min and should be titrated down slowly while the patient is monitored for return of symptoms.

94. When evaluating the 12-lead ECG of a patient recently admitted, the nurse notes: S-T elevation in leads II, III, and aVF; large Q waves in leads II, III, and aVF; and S-T depression in leads I and aVL. The nurse should suspect this is evidence that the patient has a(n)

    A. Normal ECG.
    B. Anterior wall MI.
    C. Subendocardial MI.
    D. Inferior wall MI.

95. Which of the following orders for a patient with an acute, uncomplicated MI should the nurse question?

    A. Heparin 5000 U. sub-q q 12 h.
    B. O₂ per nasal cannula at 3 L/min.
    C. Isoproterenol infusion at 20 μg/min.
    D. Morphine gr 1/4 I.V. push q 3 h PRN chest pain.

96. A type of pacemaker that senses the patient's intrinsic beats and fires only when the heart rate falls below a preset value is known as a(n) _____ pacemaker.

    A. Fixed-rate.
    B. Asynchronous.
    C. Demand.
    D. Triggered.

Answers to Questions from page 48

84. (**B**) Angina is a clinical condition characterized by pain occurring when myocardial cells are temporarily deprived of oxygen. It is an episodic ischemic condition that does not result in myocardial necrosis but could eventually lead to a myocardial infarction. The pathophysiological process of angina cannot be cured by pharmacologic agents such as nitrates, although these agents may be effective for terminating symptoms.

85. (**C**) This patient needs further evaluation because her symptoms are suggestive of angina. It is common for an angina patient's ECG to be normal in the absence of pain. The stress test, part of the diagnostic workup, seeks to induce and document ischemic changes consistent with angina.

86. (**D**) ECG changes suggestive of angina include S-T segment depression and T wave inversion, especially in the left precordial leads.

87. (**A**) Digoxin has positive inotropic and negative chronotropic effects. This fact, coupled with its slow onset of action, suggests that digoxin would not be a drug of choice for an acute anginal attack. Beta-adrenergic blocking agents, such as propranolol, are useful because they reduce myocardial oxygen consumption. Propranolol is rapid-acting when given intravenously. Nitroglycerin and nifedipine (a calcium channel blocker) have direct relaxation effects on smooth muscle, resulting in coronary vasodilation, which would alleviate anginal pain. Nitroglycerin can be given IV or sublingually and is rapid-acting. Nifedipine can be given sublingually for rapid effect by breaking the capsule.

88. (**A**) It is essential that the nurse caring for the anginal patient direct efforts toward patient and family education. It is appropriate to teach such things as modification of lifestyle, pathophysiology underlying angina, medications, and other therapy.

97. Functions of the atrial synchronous ventricular inhibited pacemaker (VDD) include

   A. Fixed-rate atrial pacing.
   B. Demand atrial pacing.
   C. Fixed-rate inhibition of spontaneous ventricular depolarization.
   D. Separate atrial and ventricular sensing.

98. Which pacemaker function does the distance of the pacemaker spike from preceding intrinsic beats reflect?

   A. Sensing.
   B. Firing.
   C. Capturing.
   D. Pulse interval.

99. The presence of pacemaker spikes *not* followed by QRS complexes indicates

   A. Inappropriate sensing.
   B. Failure to fire.
   C. Failure to capture.
   D. Use of a magnet.

100. A symptom often associated with pacemaker failure is

   A. Anorexia.
   B. Fever.
   C. Chest pain.
   D. Confusion.

101. The most common cause of congestive heart failure is dysfunction of the

   A. Right ventricle.
   B. Left ventricle.
   C. Right atrium.
   D. Left atrium.

Answers to Questions from page 49

89. (**B**) The pain associated with MI is constant, is more severe than angina, and is not relieved by nitrates or rest. It is located in the same areas as anginal pain and is frequently accompanied by nausea, vomiting, diaphoresis, dyspnea, anxiety, and dysrhythmias.

90. (**C**) The CPK elevates in 2–5 hours, peaks around 24 hours, and returns to normal in 2–3 days. The SGOT rises in 6–8 hours, peaks at 24–48 hours, and returns to normal in 4–8 days. The LDH rises in 6–12 hours, peaks at 48–72 hours, and returns to normal in 7–10 days. The SGPT is not considered a cardiac enzyme.

91. (**D**) Leukocytosis commonly occurs in response to myocardial injury. The WBC elevation is directly proportional to infarct size. The sedimentation rate also rises.

92. (**B**) The CPK-MB isoenzyme elevation is very specific for indicating myocardial infarction. The CPK-MM isoenzyme is specific for skeletal muscle and will elevate after anything that causes muscle trauma, such as I.M. injections. The LDH isoenzyme that is most specific for myocardial infarction is the LDH_1.

93. (**C**) Hypertrophic changes would not occur as an early, direct result of myocardial infarction. They may, however, be present in patients with previous underlying heart disease. ECG changes that would occur as a direct result of the infarction include evidence of ischemia, injury pattern, and evidence of necrosis.

102. The immediate pathophysiologic effect of left heart failure is

   A. Pulmonary vascular congestion.
   B. Hepatic vascular congestion.
   C. Pitting edema in the lower extremities.
   D. Cardiac tamponade.

103. Signs and symptoms that occur as a direct result of *right* heart failure include which one of the following?

   A. A cough with frothy sputum.
   B. An elevated CVP.
   C. Pulmonary hypertension.
   D. An elevated PCWP.

104. In questioning the CHF patient about his renal function, the nurse might expect this patient to have

   A. Anuria.
   B. Polyuria.
   C. Pyuria.
   D. Nocturia.

105. On physical examination the patient with CHF will most likely present with all the following, *except*

   A. Bradycardia.
   B. An S_3.
   C. Hepatojugular reflux.
   D. Bibasilar rales.

106. The position that most promotes optimal cardiac functioning in the CHF patient is

   A. Trendelenburg.
   B. Supine.
   C. Semi-Fowler's.
   D. Prone.

107. All of the following drugs are appropriate for treating pulmonary edema *except*

   A. Sodium bicarbonate.
   B. Digoxin.
   C. Morphine sulfate.
   D. Ethacrynic acid.

Answers to Questions from page 50

94. (**D**) These changes are indicative of inferior wall (diaphragmatic) MI. Indicative changes can be found in leads II, III, and aVF; reciprocal changes can be found in leads I and aVL. In an anterior wall MI, changes are found in leads I and aVL, and precordial leads of the anterior chest, with reciprocal changes in leads II, III, and aVF and posterior precordial leads. A subendocardial MI does not produce abnormal Q waves. S-T depression and T wave inversion are seen in epicardial leads over the infarct, and reciprocal changes can be seen in opposite leads.

95. (**C**) Isoproterenol has potent inotropic and chronotropic effects that result in increased myocardial oxygen demand and consumption. This agent could extend infarction size in an MI patient but might be used in small doses (up to 5 μg/min) if cardiac output is severely compromised. Prophylactic anticoagulation is useful for preventing thromboembolism. Oxygen therapy and narcotic analgesics are both appropriate forms of therapy.

96. (**C**) A demand pacemaker is described. Fixed-rate or asynchronous pacemakers fire at a preset rate without regard to intrinsic electrical activity. A demand pacemaker may be temporarily made asynchronous for the purpose of evaluating pacemaker function by placing a magnet over the generator. This technique is used when the patient is overriding the pacemaker and no pacemaker spikes are seen on ECG.

108. Which of the following electrolyte disorders is the most serious for the patient taking digoxin?

   A. Hypernatremia.
   B. Hyponatremia.
   C. Hyperkalemia.
   D. Hypokalemia.

109. Dietary teaching for the patient in CHF should involve encouraging a diet that is

   A. Low in cholesterol.
   B. Calorie-restricted.
   C. Sodium-restricted.
   D. Low in potassium.

110. A 22-year-old victim of a motorcycle accident suffered nonpenetrating chest trauma. On initial assessment, the nurse notes pleuritic-type chest pain, tachycardia, cyanosis, and muffled heart sounds. These findings are suggestive of

   A. Unilateral pneumothorax.
   B. Pericardial effusion with tamponade.
   C. Rupture of the aorta.
   D. Pneumonia.

111. A paradoxical pulse is most accurately detected by

   A. Inspection of the apical impulse.
   B. Auscultation of the blood pressure.
   C. Palpation of the radial pulse.
   D. Percussion of the cardiac borders.

112. To reduce anxiety in a patient scheduled for pericardiocentesis, the nurse should

   A. Completely sedate the patient.
   B. Give a detailed description of the procedure and its complications.
   C. Restrict visitors and leave the patient alone.
   D. Ensure a quiet, relaxed environment while providing care.

113. A diagnosis of hypertensive crisis indicates the presence of

   A. Pressures capable of vascular necrosis.
   B. Irreversible neurologic symptoms.
   C. Significant renal damage.
   D. Comatose state.

Answers to Questions from page 51

97. **(D)** The atrial synchronous ventricular inhibited pacemaker coordinates activity of both the atria and the ventricles. It senses the intrinsic activity of the atria and the ventricles and stimulates only the ventricle. For instance, if an impulse fails to arise from either the atria or ventricles, the atria are stimulated. If a spontaneous atrial impulse stimulates the ventricles, the artificial ventricular pacemaker is suppressed. If the atrial impulse does not result in ventricular stimulation, the ventricular stimulation comes from the pacemaker. The hemodynamic significance of coordinated atrial and ventricular pacing is the return of atrial kick. Another type of pacemaker that coordinates atrial and ventricular pacing is the atrial triggered pacemaker (VAT). In this device the normal atrial impulse, via the generator, triggers the ventricular pacemaker.

98. **(A)** In evaluation of a pacemaker rhythm strip for appropriate sensing, the distance from the spike to the QRS of the intrinsic beat should be the same as, or greater than the other spike-to-spike intervals. The occurrence of spikes within or immediately following the intrinsic complex usually indicates inappropriate sensing. Remember that this would not be an abnormal finding with a pacemaker that is fixed-rate, or if a magnet is being used during the strip.

99. **(C)** The presence of pacemaker spikes that do not result in ventricular depolarization is indicative of loss of capture. It may be a normal finding if a magnet is being used and the spike occurs during the refractory period of the intrinsic beat.

100. **(D)** Symptoms of pacemaker failure are all related to decreased cardiac output. Extreme fatigue, confusion, dizziness, black-outs, and slow pulse are typically seen. Symptoms of congestive heart failure may also be present.

101. **(B)** Congestive heart failure most often occurs when a diseased left ventricle loses its pumping effectiveness. Left heart failure often eventually results in right heart failure as well.

114. Signs and symptoms of hypertensive crisis include all of the following *except*

    A. Altered level of consciousness.
    B. Nystagmus.
    C. Frontal headache.
    D. Prominent apical impulse.

115. Symptoms of hypertensive encephalopathy result from

    A. Cerebral vasoconstriction.
    B. Cerebral hyperperfusion.
    C. Overstimulation of baroreceptors.
    D. Excessive levels of angiotensin II.

116. Besides blood pressure, the most critical information for the nurse to obtain on admission of a patient with hypertensive crisis is

    A. Body weight.
    B. Renal function tests.
    C. Baseline neurologic assessment.
    D. Patient history.

117. The valves most often affected by endocarditis are the

    A. Mitral and aortic valves.
    B. Mitral and tricuspid valves.
    C. Pulmonic and tricuspid valves.
    D. Pulmonic and aortic valves.

118. The signs and symptoms of endocarditis are related to all the following *except*

    A. Embolization.
    B. Cardiac involvement.
    C. Infection.
    D. Liver involvement.

| **Answers to Questions from page 52** |

102. (**A**) As the left ventricle becomes more distended, the pressure backs up through the pulmonary veins that empty into the left ventricle. As this process continues, pressure and congestion occur throughout the heart and circulatory system.

103. (**B**) In the presence of right heart failure, symptoms would result from retrograde pressure escalation. These would include such things as an elevated right atrial pressure (CVP), hepatomegaly, splenomegaly, dependent pitting edema, and jugular venous distention. Pulmonary symptoms are most often the direct effect of left heart failure.

104. (**D**) Although the patient in congestive heart failure is frequently oliguric, nocturia may occur because of improved renal perfusion at rest. The CHF patient would not be expected to have a total absence of urinary output, excessive urinary output, or pus in the urine.

105. (**A**) In CHF, the heart attempts to compensate for reduced cardiac output through tachycardia. Other physical examination findings may include an S_3, hepatojugular reflux, bibasilar rales, neck vein distention, and dependent edema.

106. (**C**) Placing the CHF patient in a semi-Fowler's position reduces venous return to the heart, lowers the diaphragm, and allows for greater lung expansion, thereby improving oxygenation. Trendelenburg, supine, and prone positions would compound the problem by increasing venous return to the heart and inhibiting maximal ventilatory function.

107. (**A**) Although patients in pulmonary edema develop respiratory acidosis, therapy involves oxygen at a high FI_2O and agents aimed at correcting the underlying problem. The sodium contained in sodium bicarbonate may aggravate the edema.

119. Cardiomyopathy may be defined as a broad category of

    A. Diseases of the pericardium.
    B. Cardiac anomalies of genetic origin.
    C. Nonprogressive cardiac disorders.
    D. Diseases of the myocardium.

120. Findings consistent with cardiomyopathy include

    A. Decreased cardiac output.
    B. Absence of precordial impulses.
    C. Decreased left atrial pressure.
    D. Decreased LVED volume.

121. Which of the following drugs would a prudent nurse question before administering to a patient with decompensated cardiomyopathy?

    A. Digitalis.
    B. Furosemide.
    C. Heparin.
    D. Propranolol.

122. The initial result of chronic mitral insufficiency is

    A. Left atrial enlargement.
    B. Severe pulmonary congestion.
    C. Left ventricular enlargement.
    D. Right heart failure.

123. You would expect the murmur associated with mitral insufficiency to be a

    A. Holosystolic murmur.
    B. Systolic ejection murmur.
    C. Protodiastolic murmur.
    D. Presystolic murmur.

124. In a valvular stenosis, the valve leaflets

    A. Atrophy and tear.
    B. Rupture.
    C. Become edematous.
    D. Calcify and immobilize.

Answers to Questions from page 53

108. (**D**) Digoxin may reach toxic levels in the hypokalemic patient. Because cardiac glycosides are frequently given concomitantly with diuretics, it is essential that the nurse monitor potassium levels and obtain an order for potassium supplement as necessary.

109. (**C**) CHF patients should be encouraged to restrict their sodium intake. Since many patients are receiving diuretics, they should also be encouraged to eat foods high in potassium.

110. (**B**) Chest trauma can result in pericarditis accompanied by effusion of fluid into the pericardial sac. This condition results in muffled heart sounds, an elevated central venous pressure, and hypotension. The resulting symptoms may include cyanosis and reflex tachycardia.

111. (**B**) When using a sphygmomanometer to detect a paradoxical pulse, one notes the reading at which systolic sounds are first heard. If systolic sounds abruptly cease, the reading at which they resume is noted. A difference of 10 mm Hg or greater indicates pulsus paradoxus. This phenomenon correlates with inspiration. It is virtually always present in cardiac tamponade and can also be indicative of constrictive pericardial disease or severe obstructive lung disease.

112. (**D**) The nurse should provide a quiet, relaxed environment while providing care for this anxious patient. It is appropriate to explain procedures to the patient; however, explanations should be brief and simple to avoid escalating the patient's anxiety.

113. (**A**) By definition, hypertensive crisis is the elevation of blood pressure to levels capable of vascular necrosis. If the condition is not resolved, damage to vessels (especially renal and retinal) may occur.

125. Which of the following chambers is *least* likely to be adversely affected in a patient with mitral stenosis?

    A. Left atrium.
    B. Right atrium.
    C. Left ventricle.
    D. Right ventricle.

126. Severe aortic insufficiency is more likely to be accompanied by all of the following *except*

    A. Diminished left ventricular end diastolic pressure.
    B. A reduction in diastolic pressure.
    C. Anginal pain.
    D. A decrescendo diastolic murmur.

127. Which of the following statements regarding aortic stenosis is *true*?

    A. It is always an acquired condition.
    B. It results in decreased afterload.
    C. It increases the ejection fraction.
    D. It results in left heart failure.

128. In aortic stenosis, the diagnostic triad that indicates the necessity of prompt valvular replacement is angina, exertional dyspnea, and

    A. Syncope.
    B. Renal failure.
    C. Widening pulse pressure.
    D. Presence of an S_3.

129. In uncomplicated atrial septal defect, which structure would *not* be expected to enlarge?

    A. Right atrium (RA).
    B. Right ventricle (RV).
    C. Left ventricle (LV).
    D. Pulmonary arteries.

130. The atrial septal defect site most likely to involve conduction abnormalities is

    A. Foramen ovale.
    B. Ostium primum.
    C. Ostium secundum.
    D. Sinus venosus.

Answers to Questions from page 54

114. (**B**) Presentation in hypertensive crisis may range from relatively asymptomatic to dramatic. Symptoms frequently seen include irritability, headache (usually frontal), confusion, seizures, and visual disturbances such as transient blindness or blurring. Level of consciousness may range from lethargy to coma. Prominent apical impulse is associated with hypertension but does not signal crisis.

115. (**B**) A mechanism of autoregulation exists to regulate cerebral perfusion. Vasodilation occurs in response to decreased pressure. In severe pressure elevation, this mechanism may fail, allowing perfusion at extremely high pressure. This may cause leakage of fluid out of the vessel and consequent cerebral edema and symptoms of hypertensive encephalopathy.

116. (**C**) In hypertensive crisis, the patient's condition may rapidly deteriorate. These changes may be detected by careful neurologic monitoring. The baseline neurologic assessment should be made immediately upon admission as a reference point for the immediate emergency management of hypertensive crisis.

117. (**A**) The valves most often affected by endocarditis are the mitral and aortic valves. Endocarditis is an inflammatory process that frequently involves accumulation of friable vegetations on valve leaflets, resulting in valvular incompetence.

118. (**D**) Signs and symptoms of endocarditis are primarily related to infection, embolization, and cardiac involvement. Embolization of infective vegetations can cause infarctions in the spleen, lungs, brain, kidneys, and coronary arteries.

131. In uncomplicated VSD, which alteration in oxygen concentration would occur?

   A. Increase in oxygen saturation or content of right ventricle.
   B. Decrease in oxygen saturation or content of right ventricle.
   C. Increase in oxygen saturation or content of left ventricle.
   D. Decrease in oxygen saturation or content of left ventricle.

132. In VSD, right-to-left shunting may occur secondary to

   A. Increased systemic vascular resistance.
   B. Increased pulmonary vascular resistance.
   C. Right ventricular enlargement.
   D. Left ventricular enlargement.

133. The most common congenital heart defect is

   A. Atrial septal defect.
   B. Ventricular septal defect.
   C. Patent ductus arteriosus.
   D. Coarctation of the aorta.

134. Increased pulmonary vascular resistance is reflected by hypertrophy of the

   A. Right ventricle.
   B. Left ventricle.
   C. Left atria.
   D. Aorta.

135. One finding associated with left-to-right shunts is

   A. Cyanosis.
   B. Bradycardia.
   C. Frequent respiratory infections.
   D. Syncope.

136. On physical assessment, you note that the patient's brachial blood pressure significantly exceeds the popliteal pressure. This finding is consistent with which congenital heart defect?

   A. Atrial septal defect.
   B. Ventricular septal defect.
   C. Patent ductus arteriosus.
   D. Coarctation of aorta.

Answers to Questions from page 55

119. (**D**) *Cardiomyopathy* designates a broad category of diseases of the myocardium. There are many different classification systems utilizing pathology or etiology. Some texts differentiate between myocardial diseases that are inflammatory (myocarditis) and those that are noninflammatory. Examples of classifications by pathology are congestive, restrictive, and idiopathic hypertrophic cardiomyopathy.

120. (**A**) Congestive heart failure, right and left, is associated with virtually all cardiomyopathies. Common symptoms may include decreased cardiac output, compensatory tachycardia, exaggeration of precordial impulse, elevated LVED, LA, and PA pressures, pulmonary and systemic congestion, dyspnea, and orthopnea.

121. (**D**) Digitalis and diuretics are often given to patients with cardiomyopathy to treat or prevent heart failure. Owing to the increased risk of systemic and pulmonary emboli, anticoagulant therapy may also be used. Because of its negative inotropic effect, propranolol would not likely be used.

122. (**C**) Because of incompetent valve closure, blood is regurgitated back into the left atrium with each ventricular contraction. This condition may reduce forward cardiac output and ultimately result in left ventricular enlargement. Because the left ventricle eventually fails, left atrial enlargement and pulmonary congestion may also ensue.

123. (**A**) Mitral insufficiency is accompanied by a holosystolic murmur. During systole, the ventricles are ejecting blood; while the left ventricle ejects blood into the aorta, blood is also regurgitating into the left atrium through the incompetent valve. During diastole, the incompetent valve allows normal left atrial emptying into the left ventricle.

124. (**D**) A stenotic valve occurs as a result of progressive fibrosis and calcification, which cause immobilization of the valve leaflets and narrowing of the valve orifice.

137. A common finding in *all* types of shock is

    A. Inadequate tissue perfusion.
    B. Diminished blood volume.
    C. Pulmonary congestion.
    D. Splanchnic congestion.

138. Hormonal responses to shock may include all *except*

    A. Increased secretion of norepinephrine.
    B. Increased secretion of aldosterone.
    C. Inhibition of renin.
    D. Release of antidiuretic hormone (ADH).

139. An indication that compensatory response mechanisms for shock are failing includes

    A. Increased heart rate.
    B. Decreased urine output.
    C. Decreased urine sodium.
    D. Pooling of blood in periphery.

140. Compensatory cardiovascular responses to shock include

    A. Constriction of coronary vessels.
    B. Peripheral vasodilation.
    C. Tachycardia.
    D. Decreased myocardial contractile force.

141. Compensatory renal responses to shock include

    A. Increased urine output.
    B. Increased glomerular filtration.
    C. Increased renal blood flow.
    D. Increased retention of sodium.

142. Which of the following most strongly suggests hypovolemia as the etiology of shock?

    A. Increased CVP.
    B. Elevated hematocrit.
    C. Increased LVEDP.
    D. Elevated serum potassium.

Answers to Questions from page 56

125. **(C)** The stenotic mitral valve does not allow adequate left atrial emptying. Left atrial hypertrophy and eventually right heart failure occur because of the retrograde pressure.

126. **(A)** In aortic insufficiency, there is regurgitation of blood back into the left ventricle during diastole. Volume overload of the left ventricle causes an elevation of left ventricular end diastolic pressure. The compromised cardiac output results in angina. This valvular defect is also characterized by an elevation in systolic blood pressure, a reduction in diastolic pressure, and a decrescendo diastolic murmur.

127. **(D)** Aortic stenosis eventually results in left heart failure because of inadequate left ventricular emptying. Aortic stenosis can be congenital or acquired, and causes increased afterload and decreased ejection fraction.

128. **(A)** The brain is very sensitive to hypoxemia; the occurrence of syncope would be indicative of the heart's inability to provide adequate cerebral perfusion. The presence of syncope, angina, and exertional dyspnea indicates the need for prompt valvular replacement.

129. **(C)** In atrial septal defects not complicated by pulmonary hypertension and ventricular hypertrophy, some blood flows from the left atrium back into the RA. This recirculation of blood causes the RA and RV to enlarge. The major pulmonary arteries also dilate.

130. **(B)** Ostium primum defects are classified as endocardial cushion defects. Possibly because of its site in the inferior atrial septum, this defect is associated with conduction abnormalities such as left axis deviation and left anterior hemiblock.

143. Microcirculatory changes associated with prolonged ischemia occur in response to release of

    A. Histamine.
    B. Vasopressin.
    C. Proteolytic enzymes.
    D. Lactase.

144. The type of shock most likely to be iatrogenic is

    A. Hypovolemic.
    B. Neurogenic.
    C. Cardiogenic.
    D. Septic.

145. Inability of the heart to meet the oxygen demands of the tissue describes which type of shock?

    A. Hypovolemic.
    B. Septic.
    C. Neurogenic.
    D. Cardiogenic.

146. The normal range for blood lactate levels is

    A. 0–4 mg/dl.
    B. 6–16 mg/dl.
    C. 18–28 mg/dl.
    D. 20–40 mg/dl.

147. While caring for a patient in septic shock, you note blood oozing from a puncture site. A prudent nurse would suspect

    A. Traumatic venipuncture.
    B. Hypoalbuminemia.
    C. Disseminated intravascular coagulation (DIC).
    D. Inadequate arterial pressure.

148. Administration of vasopressors would *least* benefit which type of shock?

    A. Hypovolemic.
    B. Neurogenic.
    C. Cardiogenic.
    D. Septic.

Answers to Questions from page 57

131. (**A**) In uncomplicated VSD, a left-to-right shunt exists. Because no mixing occurs in the left ventricle, its oxygen concentration does not change. The shunting of oxygenated blood into the right ventricle would increase the oxygen concentration of blood in that chamber.

132. (**B**) Shunting of blood from the left ventricle results in an increased pulmonary blood flow and, eventually, in increased pulmonary vascular resistance. When the right ventricle must generate more pressure than the left to eject, blood is shunted from right to left.

133. (**B**) VSD is the most common congenital heart defect, accounting for 25% of all congenital heart defects. VSD is followed in frequency by patent ductus arteriosus and coarctation of the aorta.

134. (**A**) As pulmonary vascular resistance increases, the right ventricle must work harder to empty. This increased work load results in right ventricular enlargement.

135. (**C**) Frequent respiratory infections are associated with congenital cardiac abnormalities accompanied by left-to-right shunts. They occur as a result of increased pulmonary blood volume. The increased blood flow elevates hydrostatic pressure, allowing transudation of fluid in the pulmonary capillaries.

136. (**D**) In coarctation, the restriction frequently occurs distal to the left subclavian artery. Restriction at this site causes the upper extremities to be perfused at higher than normal pressures. The blood supply to the lower extremities must pass through the coarctation, resulting in decreased pressure.

149. The type of shock associated with sudden onset of severe respiratory distress is

   A. Neurogenic.
   B. Septic.
   C. Cardiogenic.
   D. Anaphylactic.

137. (**A**) In all types of shock there is inadequate tissue perfusion. Each of the other symptoms may be found in one type of shock but not another. For example, diminished blood volume is found in hypovolemic shock but not in neurogenic shock.

138. (**C**) Baroreceptor reflex causes sympathetic stimulation that results in increased secretion of epinephrine and norepinephrine. Reduced renal perfusion pressure activates the renin-angiotensin system. Increased angiotensin II stimulates release of aldosterone. Release of ADH results in water retention in the distal tubules.

139. (**D**) Initially the heart rate and force of contraction increase in response to decreased blood pressure. Vasoconstriction shunts blood from the periphery to the vital organs. Kidneys retain sodium and water in response to decreased renal arterial pressure. When the condition persists and these mechanisms fail, peripheral vessels dilate, resulting in peripheral and splanchnic pooling.

140. (**C**) In response to a decrease in mean arterial pressure, the sympathetic nervous system triggers several physiologic responses. These include increasing the rate and force of myocardial contraction and peripheral vasoconstriction. Coronary arteries dilate to meet the higher myocardial oxygen demands associated with greater heart rate and contractile force.

141. (**D**) As a result of vasoconstriction, renal blood flow and glomerular filtration are decreased. Reduction of renal blood flow and stimulation of the renin-angiotensin system cause an increase in reabsorption of sodium and water, thereby decreasing urine output.

142. (**B**) In hypovolemic shock, CVP, cardiac output, PAP, and LVEDP are decreased. Elevated hematocrit suggest hemoconcentration. Serum potassium rises because renal and tissue perfusion is diminished.

150. The drug most appropriate for acute anaphylaxis is

    A. Atropine.
    B. Calcium chloride.
    C. Epinephrine.
    D. Phenobarbital.

Answers to Questions from page 59

143. (**A**) Histamine is released in response to cellular injury that occurs from prolonged ischemia. Microcirculatory changes that occur in response to histamine include endothelial swelling and separation, which allow passage of fluid and particles through the capillary membranes.

144. (**D**) Septic shock may occur in response to organisms acquired during hospitalization. Frequency of invasive procedures also predisposes patients to infection. Foley catheterization resulting in urinary tract infection is another potential cause of septic shock.

145. (**D**) *Cardiogenic shock* is inadequate tissue perfusion due to inadequate cardiac pumping. In the other types of shock, the decrease in cardiac output is secondary to another process. Some of the causes of cardiogenic shock are MI, cardiac tamponade, pulmonary embolus, and CHF.

146. (**B**) Normal blood lactate levels range from 6–16 mg/dl. In the absence of adequate tissue oxygen, anaerobic metabolism occurs, resulting in a build-up of lactic acid. Marked elevations in blood lactate level generally occur late in the shock syndrome.

147. (**C**) DIC may complicate sepsis as well as other types of shock. It is characterized by generalized bleeding. Symptoms include oozing from puncture sites, prolonged clotting times, petechiae, hematomas, and acral cyanosis.

148. (**A**) In hypovolemic shock, there is a decrease in circulating blood volume. Sympathetic response to hypotension is usually normal; therefore, vasopressors have limited effectiveness. Volume replacement is the recommended management of hypovolemic shock.

| Answers to Questions from page 60 | Answers to Questions from page 61 |

149. (**A**) Anaphylactic shock is associated with sudden onset of severe respiratory distress. Laryngeal edema and bronchospasm are often seen. Respiratory stridor and prominent wheezes accompany respiratory embarrassment.

150. (**C**) Anaphylaxis is an acute allergic response. Onset is usually rapid after contact with the stimulus. One common cause of anaphylactic response is administration of penicillin. Epinephrine relaxes bronchospasm, controls histamine release, and increases cardiac output.

Bibliography

American Association of Critical-Care Nurses: Core Curriculum For Critical Care Nursing, 3rd ed. W. B. Saunders Co., Philadelphia, 1985.
Presented in a nursing process approach utilizing outline format. Includes salient points relevant to each major body system. Good text for delineating essential information for a holistic understanding of the human body. Appropriate for critical care practitioners, educators, and students.

Bates, B.: A Guide To Physical Examination, 3rd ed. J. B. Lippincott Co., Philadelphia, 1983.
Provides a good description of normal physical findings. Presents physical assessment techniques in a basic, easily understood manner. Provides numerous helpful illustrations.

Brunner, L. S., and Suddarth, D. S.: The Lippincott Manual of Nursing Practice, 3rd ed. J. B. Lippincott Co., Philadelphia, 1982.
Content is presented in numerical format and relates to various procedures and disease states. Includes nursing management and goals but is limited in medical management. Critical information is printed throughout text in colored "nursing alert" boxes.

Braunwald, E.: Heart Disease: A Texbook of Cardiovascular Medicine, 2nd ed. Volume I. W. B. Saunders Co., Philadelphia, 1984.
A complex text that addresses in detail numerous cardiovascular disorders. Devotes entire chapters to many diagnostic procedures. Explains principles, techniques, interpretation, and risks of diagnostic procedures.

Budassi, S. A., and Barber, J. M.: Emergency Nursing Principles and Practice. C. V. Mosby Co., St. Louis, 1981.
Deals thoroughly with acute intervention appropriate in all types of emergency situations. Includes brief discussion of pathophysiology. Numerous illustrations enhance content. Excellent comprehensive appendices, such as legal standards, pharmacology, and laboratory values.

Hudak, C. M., Lohr, T., and Gallo, B. M.: Critical Care Nursing, 3rd ed. J. B. Lippincott Co., Philadelphia, 1982.
A critical care text that summarizes essential information for understanding conditions requiring acute interventions. Easy to read and understand.

Hurst, J. W., Logue, R. B., Schlant, R. C., Weyer, N. K.: The Heart, 4th ed. McGraw-Hill Book Co., New York, 1978.
Complete reference text of cardiology. Presents very complex information in easily understood manner. An essential cardiology resource book.

Kinney, M. R., Dear, C. B., Packa, D. R., and Voorman, D. M. (eds.): AACN's Clinical Reference for Critical Care Nursing. McGraw-Hill Book Co., New York, 1981.
A very comprehensive text for critical care nurses. Separate chapters deal with physiology and pathophysiology of body systems.

Larson, E. L., and Vazquez, M. (eds.): Critical Care Nursing, W. B. Saunders Co., Philadelphia, 1983.
An excellent quick reference for critical care nurses. Addresses wide variety of clinical disorders, including an overview of the disorder, pertinent assessment, and priorities of nursing management. Excellent appendices for quick reference.

Marriott, H. L.: Practical Electrocardiography, 7th ed. Williams & Wilkins Co., Baltimore, 1983.
An excellent, comprehensive text written in a conversational manner. All aspects of electrocardiography are presented; may, however, prove a bit too advanced for the beginning practitioner.

McGurn, W. C.: People With Cardiac Problems: Nursing Concepts. J. B. Lippincott Co., Philadelphia, 1981.
Very good text for nurses caring for cardiac patients. Deals with biophysical and psychosocial aspects of cardiac illnesses. Extensive information necessary for patient education and rehabilitation included.

McIntyre, K. M., and Lewis, A. J. (eds.): Textbook of Advanced Cardiac Life Support. American Heart Association, Dallas, 1981.
Concisely summarizes critical concepts of advanced life support. Information is all current, documented throughout with recent research findings.

Meltzer, L. E., Pinneo, R., and Kitchell, J. R.: Intensive Coronary Care: A Manual For Nurses, 4th ed. Robert J. Brady Co., Bowie, Maryland, 1983.
A good text for understanding cardiac electrophysiology. Dysrhythmias are presented in a logical, easily understood manner. Appendices include sections on cardiac drugs and exercises in dysrhythmia interpretation.

Petersdorf, R. G., Adams, R. D., Braunwald, E., Isselbacher, K. J., and Wilson, J. D. (eds.): Harrison's Principles of Internal Medicine, 10th ed. McGraw-Hill Book Co., New York, 1983.
An excellent resource containing exhaustive content relative to internal medicine. Provides a good understanding of pathophysiological basis for diseases as well as appropriate treatment.

Rose, D. B.: Clinical Physiology of Acid, Base and Electrolyte Disorders. McGraw-Hill Book Co., St. Louis, 1977.
Deals in depth with acid-base and electrolyte physiology and pathophysiology. Throughout the text, clinical situations are given, providing opportunities to apply concepts that are presented. Extremely comprehensive list of references for each chapter.

Sanderson, R. G., and Kurth, C. L.: The Cardiac Patient: A Comprehensive Approach, 2nd ed. W. B. Saunders Co., Philadelphia, 1983.
Deals with pathophysiology of cardiac conditions. Includes the most current diagnostic procedures and therapeutic techniques. Contains a useful chapter on cardiac rehabilitation.

Thompson, J. M., and Bowers, A. C.: Clinical Manual of Health Assessment. C. V. Mosby Co., St. Louis, 1980.
Comprehensive physical assessment guide that gives good descriptions of normals with descriptions and illustrations of deviations from normal. Organized utilizing a systems approach. Each system discussion ends with a post-test for self-assessment.

Tilkian, A. G., and Conover, M. B.: Understanding Heart Sounds and Murmurs, 2nd ed. W. B. Saunders Co., Philadelphia, 1984.
An easily understood paperback text that presents heart sounds in a basic yet thorough manner. In addition to normal and abnormal heart sounds, clinical techniques that facilitate detection of abnormalities are presented. A glossary of related terms is also included. Excellent reference for studying cardiac auscultation.

Wenger, N. K., Hurst, J. W., and McIntyre, M. C.: Cardiology for Nurses. McGraw-Hill Book Co., St. Louis, 1980.
Cardiology reference text written from a nursing perspective. Brief overview of related physiology, pathophysiology, and etiology of each condition is presented. The remainder of information for each topic is presented in care plan fashion: data base (history and physical) and plan of care. Plan of care is divided into diagnostic, therapeutic, and educational goals. Includes x-rays and ECGs for many topics. Excellent reference for nurses.

3 □ THE NEUROLOGIC SYSTEM

NANCY M. HOLLOWAY

1. An example of a supratentorial structure is the:

   A. Spinal cord.
   B. Cerebellum.
   C. Corpus callosum.
   D. Medulla.

2. A patient with an inability to localize touch would be most likely to have a lesion of which lobe of the brain?

   A. Temporal.
   B. Parietal.
   C. Occipital.
   D. Frontal.

3. Which of the following statements correctly describes the basal ganglia?

   A. They are a major center of the pyramidal system.
   B. They are located in the frontal lobe.
   C. They regulate muscle tone and postural reflexes.
   D. Paralysis is their primary disease process.

4. An individual with a hypothalamic disorder would most likely have a problem with which of the following processes?

   A. Relaying sensory information from sensory pathways.
   B. Maintaining the body's internal environment.
   C. Establishing the basic rhythmic pattern of respiration.
   D. Perceiving and interpreting auditory stimuli.

5. What is the significance of the circle of Willis?

    A. It is commonly injured in head trauma.
    B. Its disruption results in myasthenia gravis.
    C. It provides collateral cerebral circulation if one of the arteries to the brain becomes occluded.
    D. It provides collateral venous drainage if the superior sagittal sinus becomes obstructed.

6. Cerebrospinal fluid (CSF) is reabsorbed into the venous system via the:

    A. Arachnoid villi.
    B. Aqueduct of Sylvius.
    C. Foramen of Monro.
    D. Choroid plexuses.

7. Which of the following components of a neuron carries out its major metabolic functions?

    A. Axon hillock.
    B. Dendrites.
    C. Nodes of Ranvier.
    D. Cell body.

8. What is the significance of the blood-brain barrier?

    A. It limits the transmission of substances from the blood to the brain.
    B. It is thought to result from increased capillary permeability.
    C. It allows drugs to diffuse freely from the interstitial space to the intravascular space.
    D. Its disruption is rare in head-injured patients.

9. In normal neuromuscular transmission, which structure or substance limits the duration of the action potential?

   A. Synaptic cleft.
   B. Acetylcholinesterase.
   C. Serotonin.
   D. Motor end-plate.

10. Pain and temperature sensations ascend the spinal cord in which structure?

   A. Spinothalamic tract.
   B. Corticospinal tract.
   C. Extrapyramidal system.
   D. Dorsal columns.

Answers to Questions from page 65

1. (C) The tentorium cerebelli is a fold of the dura mater that separates the cerebrum (specifically, the occipital lobes) from the cerebellum. The corpus callosum, commissural fibers that connect one area of a cerebral hemisphere with its corresponding area in the other hemisphere, lies above the tentorium. The cerebellum, medulla, and spinal cord all lie below it.

2. (B) The parietal lobe is primarily responsible for sensory function, including sensory association and higher-level processing of general sensory information, e.g., two-point discrimination. The frontal lobes control higher mental functions (e.g. judgment and intellect) and voluntary motor function. The temporal lobes are responsible for hearing, speech in the dominant hemisphere, vestibular function, and some aspects of emotion and behavior. The occipital lobes are responsible for vision.

3. (C) The basal ganglia are deep cerebral structures that exert controlling influences on muscle tone, postural reflexes, and motor integration. They are a major component of the extrapyramidal system, and their primary disease process is Parkinsonism.

4. (B) The hypothalamus has multiple functions that serve to maintain the body's internal environment. Among these functions are regulation of body temperature, of body water (through secretion of antidiuretic hormone), of cardiovascular stability, of food intake, and of pituitary function. The relay of sensory information is mediated by the thalamus. Auditory associations occur in the temporal lobe. Although the hypothalamus can influence respiration indirectly (e.g., via its heat regulatory function), its role is secondary to that of the medullary respiratory center, which sets the basic pattern of respiration.

11. An example of a pure upper motor neuron lesion is:

    A. Poliomyelitis.
    B. Spinal cord injury below L_1–L_2 vertebral level.
    C. Amyotrophic lateral sclerosis.
    D. Cerebrovascular accident with spastic paralysis.

12. Physiologic responses to stimulation of the sympathetic nervous system include:

    A. Increased peristalsis.
    B. Decreased cardiac contractility.
    C. Bronchodilation.
    D. Pupillary constriction.

13. Which visual defect would be displayed by a patient with a lesion of the left optic tract?

    A. Unilateral total blindness.
    B. Bitemporal hemianopsia.
    C. Right homonymous hemianopsia.
    D. Left homonymous hemianopsia with macular sparing.

Answers to Questions from page 66

5. **(C)** The circle of Willis is a ring of blood vessels at the base of the brain that surround the pituitary stalk and optic chiasm. The anterior portion of the circle of Willis arises from the internal carotid arteries, and the posterior portion arises from the vertebral arteries. The circle itself consists of the anterior and posterior cerebral arteries and their communicating arteries. Should one of the carotid or vertebral arteries become occluded, the circle of Willis can provide collateral circulation.

6. **(A)** All of the structures named participate in the formation, circulation, and/or reabsorption of CSF. The choroid plexuses of the ventricles continually form CSF. CSF passes from the lateral ventricles through the foramen of Monro into the third ventricle and then through the aqueduct of Sylvius into the fourth ventricle. After leaving the fourth ventricle, CSF circulates around the brain in the subarachnoid space. The arachnoid villi, projections of the arachnoid layer into the superior saggital and transverse sinuses, are the pathways through which CSF is reabsorbed into the venous system.

7. **(D)** A neuron basically consists of a cell body and its extensions, the dendrites and axon. The cell body (soma) carries out the major metabolic functions. Dendrites carry impulses toward the cell body, and the axon conducts them away. The axon hillock is a thickened area of the cell body from which the axon arises. Nodes of Ranvier are found on some axons. They are periodic constrictions where the axon is not covered by a myelin sheath, and they play an important role in rapid saltatory conduction of impulses.

8. **(A)** The blood-brain barrier is a permeability phenomenon that limits the movement of substances from the brain capillaries to the cerebrospinal fluid. One mechanism involved in the barrier is decreased capillary permeability, which is thought to be due to tight junctions of the brain's endothelial cells. The barrier often is disrupted in head injury.

14. A normal consensual light reflex indicates proper functioning of which two cranial nerves?

   A. Abducens and acoustic.
   B. Ophthalmic and hypoglossal.
   C. Optic and oculomotor.
   D. Trochlear and vagal.

15. Assessment of reflexes in your 30-year-old patient reveals a Babinski sign. This datum indicates damage to the:

   A. Pyramidal tract.
   B. Cerebellum.
   C. Extrapyramidal system.
   D. Anterior spinothalamic tract.

16. A patient who sways when standing with his feet together and eyes closed (Romberg's sign) and who is unable to walk heel-to-toe would most likely have a dysfunction of which of the following areas of the neurologic system?

   A. Hypothalamic.
   B. Oculomotor.
   C. Corticospinal.
   D. Cerebellar.

17. The following values are reported for a cerebrospinal fluid (CSF) analysis: clear, colorless; 3 white blood cells per mm^3; protein 90 mg/100 ml; glucose 60 mg/100 ml. The correct interpretation would be that:

   A. This is a normal CSF report.
   B. The protein level is elevated.
   C. The presence of white blood cells indicates infection.
   D. The serum glucose probably is decreased.

18. The initial diagnostic procedure of choice in acute head trauma is:

   A. Air encephalography.
   B. Cerebral angiography.
   C. Electromyography.
   D. Computerized tomography.

Answers to Questions from page 67

9. (**B**) The *motor end-plate* is a flattened area where the nerve loses its myelin sheath and lies close to the motor fiber. The space between the end of the nerve and the motor fiber is the *synaptic cleft*. Vesicles in the nerve terminal release the neurotransmitter acetylcholine, which then diffuses across the synaptic cleft to alter the permeability of the muscle membrane and trigger an action potential. *Acetylcholinesterase* is an enzyme that breaks down acetylcholine, thus limiting the duration of the action potential. *Serotonin* is a neurotransmitter implicated in sleep behavior.

10. (**A**) The ascending spinal cord tracts carry sensory information from the periphery to the brain. Of the possible answers, two are ascending tracts: the spinothalamic tract and the dorsal columns. The *spinothalamic tract* carries pain and temperature sensations, and the *dorsal columns* convey sensations of complex sensory discrimination, touch, vibration, and joint position. The corticospinal tract and extrapyramidal system are descending structures. The *corticospinal tract* mediates voluntary movement, carrying impulses from the motor cortex down the spine. The *extrapyramidal system* consists of numerous tracts that both inhibit and facilitate motor activity, particularly muscle tone, equilibrium, and postural reflexes.

19. The nurse should be aware that a patient undergoing CT scanning or cerebral angiography with injection of contrast medium may experience all of the following except:

    A. Allergic response.
    B. Hallucinations.
    C. Fluid overload.
    D. Osmotic diuresis.

20. Consciousness depends on the interaction between:

    A. The reticular activating system and cerebral cortex.
    B. The basal ganglia and hypothalamus.
    C. The pyramidal and extrapyramidal systems.
    D. The dorsal columns and dermatomes.

21. A critical care nurse is told that a head-injured patient has a Glasgow Coma Score of 8. The nurse knows that all of the following abilities were assessed except:

    A. Eye opening.
    B. Vital signs.
    C. Motor response.
    D. Verbal response.

Answers to Questions from page 68

11. (**D**) A lower motor neuron consists of the anterior horn cell of the spinal cord and its efferent motor neuron. It is sometimes referred to as the "final common pathway" for motor impulses. An upper motor neuron is one that both originates and ends in the central nervous system, i.e., any neuron that provides input to the anterior horn cell of the spinal cord and thus influences the "final common pathway." The major upper motor neuron structures are the cerebral cortex (especially the corticospinal tract), cerebellum, basal ganglia, and reticular neurons. Poliomyelitis destroys anterior horn cells, whereas a spinal cord injury below L_1–L_2 (where the cord itself ends) affects only nerve fibers that have already exited from the spinal cord. Amyotrophic lateral sclerosis can cause degeneration of the lower motor neuron as well as the upper motor neuron. A cerebrovascular accident may occur in the cerebral cortex, thus affecting the upper motor neuron and producing spastic paralysis.

12. (**C**) Sympathetic autonomic nervous system stimulation results in the "fight or flight" response. The heart rate accelerates, cardiac contractility increases, pupils dilate (to better see the "enemy"), and bronchi dilate (to allow increased air intake). Peristalsis is decreased during sympathetic stimulation.

13. (**C**) Fibers from the nasal halves of the retinas cross at the optic chiasm and join uncrossed fibers from the temporal halves of the retinas to form the optic tracts. A lesion of the left optic tract therefore causes damage to transmission of sight by the left half of the retinas. Since these halves perceive images in the right halves of the visual fields, the patient develops right homonymous hemianopsia. Unilateral blindness results from damage to the eye, retina, or optic nerve. Bitemporal hemianopsia results from a lesion of the center of the optic chiasm (a rare occurrence). Hemianopsia with macular sparing results from a lesion of the geniculocalcarine tract.

22. The development of unequal pupils in a patient can indicate a life-threatening disorder. Which of the following disorders would be the most life-threatening cause of the inequality?

   A. Tentorial herniation disrupting oculomotor nerve fibers.
   B. Cervical spine injury disrupting sympathetic pathways.
   C. Major cerebral hemorrhage in the midbrain.
   D. Major trigeminal nerve damage.

23. Which of the following accurately describes the doll's eyes test (for oculocephalic reflex)?

   A. It is important to perform when cervical spine injury is suspected.
   B. Its result is normal if the eyes turn in the same direction as the head.
   C. The response is elicited by injecting iced water into the ears.
   D. It is a test to evaluate brainstem integrity.

24. Your patient displays a respiratory pattern that alternately crescendos to hyperpnea and decrescendos to apnea. The correct term for this respiratory pattern is:

   A. Post-hyperventilation apnea.
   B. Cheyne-Stokes respiration.
   C. Neurogenic hyperventilation.
   D. Biot's breathing.

Answers to Questions from page 69

14. **(C)** The consensual light reflex occurs when light stimulation of one eye provokes constriction of the other pupil. It indicates that stimuli are being perceived by the optic nerve and transmitted to the oculomotor nerves, which cause constriction of both the stimulated pupil (direct light reflex) and the other pupil (consensual light reflex).

15. **(A)** A Babinski sign is dorsiflexion of the big toe, with or without fanning of the other toes, when a sharp object is used to stroke up the lateral sole and across the ball of the foot. It indicates damage to the pyramidal portion of the motor cortex (upper motor neuron injury). The Babinski sign is normal in children up to 2 years old.

16. **(D)** A patient who presents in this manner is displaying an inability to coordinate muscle groups. Muscle group coordination, necessary for smooth movements, is controlled by the cerebellum. Because many conditions may cause gait disturbances and because vestibular dysfunction also may elicit Romberg's sign, this patient does not necessarily have cerebellar dysfunction. However, of the four possible choices, D is the most correct.

17. **(B)** CSF normally is clear and colorless and contains 0–6 white blood cells per mm^3. The glucose level varies with the serum glucose, averaging about 60% of the serum value; it usually is 50–75 mg/100 ml. The protein level varies with the CSF sampling site but usually does not exceed 45 mg/100 ml. Protein elevations occur in many disorders, most commonly meningitis.

18. **(D)** Computerized tomography (CT scan) is a sensitive, painless diagnostic procedure that can provide an immediate scan printout in emergency situations, such as the need for detection of a rapidly expanding intracranial mass. It has replaced air encephalography and cerebral angiography as the primary diagnostic procedure for identification of intracranial masses. Electromyography, the recording of muscle electrical potentials, is used in the diagnosis of muscle disorders.

25. What level of lesion correlates with the respiratory pattern described in question 24?

    A. Pontine.
    B. Forebrain.
    C. Cerebral hemispheres.
    D. Medulla.

26. Which of the following is the most sensitive indicator of increasing ICP?

    A. Blood pressure.
    B. Level of consciousness.
    C. Cushing's reflex.
    D. Pulse volume.

27. A common cause of hypoxemia in the CNS-injured patient is:

    A. Pulmonary shunt.
    B. Central neurogenic hyperventilation.
    C. Decreased capillary permeability.
    D. Vomiting.

28. A patient with a skull fracture and bilateral femoral fractures becomes confused and develops petechiae. These findings suggest the development of which of the following complications?

    A. Psychogenic invalidism.
    B. Ventricular dysrhythmia.
    C. Fat embolism.
    D. Acute tubular necrosis.

29. The nurse should be concerned about the neurosurgical patient with a blood pH above 7.5 because:

    A. The elevated Pa_{CO_2} will cause cerebral vasodilatation.
    B. A leftward shift of the oxyhemoglobin dissociation curve may impair tissue oxygen delivery.
    C. Alkalosis is associated with hyperkalemia.
    D. The reported pH probably is due to tissue hypoxia.

Answers to Questions from page 70

19. (**B**) The iodine-based contrast media may provoke an allergic response, so the nurse should ask about past reactions to contrast media and to iodine-containing foods such as soft-shelled seafood. Since the dye is hypertonic, it causes an interstitial-to-plasma fluid shift that can provoke fluid overload, particularly in patients with cardiac or renal disease. Because of the increased blood volume and renal excretion of the dye, osmotic diuresis occurs.

20. (**A**) Consciousness consists of two components: arousal (wakefulness) and cognitive functioning (content). Arousal is controlled by the reticular activating system (RAS), located in the brainstem and diencephalon. When stimulated, the RAS causes diffuse arousal of the central nervous system and specific arousal of areas of the cerebral cortex. The content of consciousness, that is, cognitive functioning, depends on the cerebral cortex. For full consciousness, therefore, the patient must have both a normally functioning RAS and reasonably intact cerebral hemispheres.

21. (**B**) The Glasgow Coma Scale evaluates three components of behavior: eye opening, best verbal response, and best motor response. It provides an objective and reliable tool to assess level of consciousness. The scores for each component are added to produce an overall score for level of consciousness. Since the score does not include vital signs, the critical care nurse would need to incorporate vital sign measurement in further patient assessment.

30. All of the following factors may be present in patients with severe cerebral ischemia. The one that makes it especially important to maintain a normal or, in some cases, even slightly hypertensive systemic blood pressure is:

    A. Loss of cerebral autoregulation.
    B. No reflow phenomenon.
    C. Vasomotor paralysis.
    D. Cytotoxic cerebral edema.

31. Patients with which of the following disorders are more likely to experience dysrhythmias?

    A. Myasthenia gravis.
    B. Guillain-Barré syndrome.
    C. Meningitis.
    D. Subarachnoid hemorrhage.

32. Which of the following laboratory findings is consistent with the syndrome of inappropriate ADH release?

    A. Serum sodium level above 145 mEq/L.
    B. Urine sodium level less than 25 mEq/L.
    C. Serum osmolality below 275 mOsm/kg.
    D. Serum osmolality greater than urine osmolality.

33. Which of the following statements correctly describes intracranial dynamics?

    A. A patient's response to changes in intracranial pressure (ICP) is independent of his position on the cerebral compliance curve.
    B. Under normal circumstances, cerebral autoregulation maintains a constant cerebral blood flow over a wide range of systemic arterial pressures.
    C. If systemic blood pressure remains constant, decreased ICP will cause a decrease in cerebral perfusion pressure.
    D. The Cushing reflex is an early compensatory response to increased ICP.

Answers to Questions from page 71

22. (**A**) Pupil size reflects the balance between sympathetic and parasympathetic stimulation. When transtentorial herniation occurs, disruption of the oculomotor nerve's parasympathetic fibers causes the ipsilateral pupil to dilate because of the dominant sympathetic influence. This herniation is a life-threatening emergency. When sympathetic pathways in the cervical cord are transected, the predominance of parasympathetic stimulation causes the pupil on the same side to constrict (Horner's syndrome). However, the inequality of the pupils in this setting does not indicate a life-threatening emergency. Major midbrain damage interrupts both the sympathetic and the parasympathetic pathways to the eyes, which become fixed in midposition. Damage to the trigeminal nerve will affect corneal sensation but not pupillary size.

23. (**D**) The doll's eyes test evaluates the integrity of the brainstem, specifically the connections between cranial nerves VIII (which carries vestibular sensations) and III and VI (which move the eyes medially and laterally). It is evaluated in the unconscious patient. If the reflex arcs are intact, brisk head turning to one side will produce eye movement toward the opposite side. The test should not be performed on someone with a suspected cervical spine injury. Iced-water irrigation of the ears also is used to test midbrain integrity, but the test involved is called iced-water calorics and evaluates the oculovestibular reflex.

24. (**B**) The pattern described is Cheyne-Stokes respiration. *Post-hyperventilation apnea* is apnea that occurs after deep breathing lowers the Pa_{CO_2} below normal. *Neurogenic hyperventilation* is characterized by prolonged, rapid, deep respirations. *Biot's breathing* is a totally irregular pattern of randomly occurring rapid and deep breaths.

34. A patient with which of the following arterial blood pressure (BP) and intracranial pressure (ICP) readings would have a normal cerebral perfusion pressure? All pressures are given in mm Hg.

    A. BP 145/70; ICP 5.
    B. BP 280/160; ICP 10.
    C. BP 80/50; ICP 5.
    D. BP 165/105; ICP 10.

35. A patient with an elevated ICP suddenly develops a unilaterally dilated pupil. The nurse realizes that the significance of this sign is that the patient is undergoing what pathophysiologic process?

    A. Herniation under the falx cerebri.
    B. Uncal herniation.
    C. Cerebellar tonsillar herniation.
    D. Central herniation.

36. Nursing responsibilities with intracranial pressure monitoring systems include which of the following?

    A. With an epidural monitoring system, periodically sampling CSF.
    B. With an intraventricular monitoring system, maintaining the transducer below the level of the foramen of Monro.
    C. With a subarachnoid screw, opening the system to air to zero-balance it.
    D. With an intraventricular monitoring system, maintaining patency with a continuous low-flow flush device.

37. Assuming all of the following methods are possible, one method to rapidly lower the ICP in a mechanically ventilated patient is:

    A. Hyperventilation.
    B. Suctioning the airway.
    C. Adding dead space to the ventilator tubing.
    D. Lowering the FI_{O_2}.

Answers to Questions from page 72

25. (C) Cheyne-Stokes respiration may indicate bilateral lesions of the cerebral hemispheres or basal ganglia, or metabolic problems. Pontine lesions may produce neurogenic hyperventilation, apneustic breathing, or cluster breathing; forebrain lesions may produce post-hyperventilation apnea; and medullary lesions may produce ataxic (Biot's) breathing.

26. (B) The level of consciousness is the most sensitive indicator of increasing ICP. Blood pressure and pulse are notoriously unreliable indicators of ICP. They are unpredictably associated with ICP, and when BP and pulse changes do occur, they are late. Cushing's reflex is a systolic pressure rise that exceeds the diastolic pressure rise. It is the body's "last ditch" attempt to improve cerebral perfusion in intracranial hypertension.

27. (A) There appears to be a relationship between CNS injury and hypoxemia. Although the exact mechanisms are unclear, pulmonary shunt plays a role. Central neurogenic hyperventilation is not a cause of hypoxemia; instead, it may be a manifestation. It also may result from midbrain or midpontine lesions. Increased rather than decreased capillary permeability plays a role in hypoxia via its contribution to neurogenic pulmonary edema. Vomiting does not produce hypoxia unless aspiration occurs.

28. (C) The patient's history of a long-bone fracture and petechiae strongly point to fat embolism as the cause of the confusion.

29. (B) Alkalosis shifts the oxyhemoglobin dissociation curve to the left, binding oxygen more tightly to hemoglobin so that less may be delivered to the tissues. An elevated Pa_{CO_2} is associated with acidosis rather than alkalosis. Alkalosis usually is associated with hypokalemia rather than hyperkalemia. Tissue hypoxia is likely to produce metabolic acidosis rather than an alkalosis.

38. When caring for a person with an open depressed fracture of the temporal bone, the nurse should be aware of the potential for all of the following complications *except:*

    A. Epidural hematoma.
    B. Facial paralysis.
    C. Tongue deviation.
    D. Vertigo or hearing loss.

39. Bilateral ecchymotic eyes ("owl's eyes" or "raccoon's eyes") may be seen in what type of fracture?

    A. Anterior fossa.
    B. Middle fossa.
    C. Posterior fossa.
    D. Lateral fossa.

40. A patient with CSF rhinorrhea would benefit most from nursing care that includes:

    A. Assistance with nasal packing to tamponade the leak.
    B. Insertion of a nasogastric tube to aspirate swallowed CSF.
    C. Testing the fluid with litmus paper.
    D. Administration of prophylactic antibiotics.

41. An individual with cerebral concussion would be expected to experience all but which one of the following clinical syndromes?

    A. Retrograde amnesia.
    B. 24-hour loss of consciousness.
    C. Anterograde (post-traumatic) amnesia.
    D. Post-concussion syndrome.

42. A patient is admitted to a critical care unit drowsy and with multiple fractures. The limited history available on admission is: victim of a motor vehicle accident, head struck roof of car, unconscious when the paramedics arrived but rapidly regained consciousness. In analyzing this situation, the critical care nurse realizes the patient is at greatest risk for:

    A. Subarachnoid hemorrhage.
    B. Acute subdural hematoma.
    C. Epidural hematoma.
    D. Chronic subdural hematoma.

Answers to Questions from page 73

30. **(A)** Although all four pathophysiologic processes may exist in cerebral ischemia, the one that relates specifically to the need to maintain normal or elevated systemic blood pressure is loss of cerebral autoregulation. This loss causes cerebral blood flow to vary more directly with blood pressure than normal. In certain pathologic states with markedly elevated intracranial pressure, loss of autoregulation may necessitate maintenance of systemic blood pressure in a slightly hypertensive state in order to maintain cerebral perfusion.

31. **(D)** Although dysrhythmias may occur in any neurologic patient, they are most likely to occur in subarachnoid hemorrhage, stroke, intracranial hypertension, and head trauma.

32. **(C)** The syndrome of inappropriate ADH release produces excessive water retention and hyponatremia. Serum osmolality falls below urine osmolality. In spite of the serum hyponatremia, sodium loss continues in the urine; the mechanism is unclear but may be related to sodium diuresis caused by increased blood flow through the kidneys.

33. **(B)** Although systemic arterial pressures may fluctuate widely, cerebral autoregulation maintains a constant cerebral blood flow under normal circumstances. A patient's response to increased intracranial pressure does depend on his position on the compliance curve: on the steep portion of the curve, even small volume changes can result in large pressure changes. If systemic BP remains constant, a decreased ICP will result in an improved CPP. The Cushing reflex is a late response to increased ICP.

43. An alcoholic is a prime candidate for an undetected chronic subdural hematoma because of all of the following factors *except*:

  A. Decreased clotting factors due to cirrhosis of the liver.
  B. Alcoholic dilatation of the pupils obscuring pupillary signs.
  C. Increased likelihood of a missed diagnosis due to difficulty evaluating level of consciousness in an inebriated patient.
  D. A history of frequent falls.

44. An intracerebral hematoma may result from:

  A. Fracture lacerating the middle meningeal artery.
  B. Tear of the dura mater.
  C. Polycythemia.
  D. Rupture of an intracranial aneurysm.

34. (**A**) Cerebral perfusion pressure equals mean arterial pressure minus mean intracranial pressure. Mean arterial pressure (MAP) is calculated by adding ⅓ the pulse pressure (systolic pressure minus diastolic pressure) to the diastolic pressure. The normal value for CPP is 80–90 mm Hg. Since CPP = MAP − ICP, answer A is correct.

35. (**B**) Herniation of the uncus of the temporal lobe over the edge of the tentorial opening causes compression or stretching of the oculomotor nerve on the same side as a supratentorial lesion. This compression impairs the nerve's parasympathetic fibers, so unopposed sympathetic stimulation causes the pupil to dilate. The syndromes of herniation under the falx cerebri, central herniation through the tentorial opening, and cerebellar tonsillar herniation through the foramen magnum do not produce unilateral pupillary dilatation.

36. (**C**) The monitoring system used with a subarachnoid screw must be opened to air periodically for zero-balancing. An epidural system cannot be used to sample CSF, as it does not communicate with the structure through which CSF circulates. The transducer in an intraventricular system should be maintained at the level of the foramen of Monro for accurate readings. A continuous low-flow flush device should never be connected to an intraventricular catheter because of the danger of infusing a large amount of fluid and precipitating herniation.

37. (**A**) Mechanical hyperventilation rapidly lowers the patient's Pa_{CO_2}, causing cerebral arterioles to constrict and therefore reducing cerebral blood flow and ICP. Adding deadspace would cause increased CO_2 retention, thus promoting cerebral vasodilation and increased ICP. Lowering the FI_{O_2} would promote hypoxemia, aggravating cerebral vasodilation and increased ICP. Suctioning is a noxious stimulus that raises ICP.

45. A patient who has been stabbed in the back develops lower extremity paralysis on the same side as the wound and loses pain and temperature sensations on the side of the body opposite the injury. This type of spinal cord injury is referred to as a:

   A. Total transection.
   B. Anterior cord syndrome.
   C. Central cord syndrome.
   D. Brown-Séquard syndrome.

46. A patient sustains a spinal cord injury at C_6 and remains conscious and alert. The nurse knows that, barring complications, the outcome for this patient may include retaining all of the following functional capacities *except*:

   A. Diaphragmatic breathing.
   B. Picking up objects with fingers.
   C. Reaching forward.
   D. Sitting upright with support.

Answers to Questions from page 75

38. **(C)** Fractures of the temporal bone may be associated with laceration of the middle meningeal artery, leading to an epidural hematoma. They also may be associated with damage to nearby nerves. Facial paralysis may result from damage to the seventh cranial nerve, and disturbances in hearing or equilibrium may result from damage to the eighth cranial nerve. Control of the tongue is governed by the hypoglossal or 12th cranial nerve, which should not be affected by this lesion.

39. **(A)** "Raccoon's eyes" are seen with anterior fossa fractures, owing to bleeding into the sinuses. Ecchymoses over the mastoid bone (Battle's sign) are seen with middle fossa fractures.

40. **(D)** The person with a CSF leak would benefit most from nursing care that includes administration of prophylactic antibiotics. Nasal packing is ineffective and unnecessary; the site of the dural tear may be beyond reach, and the leak usually stops spontaneously. The fluid should be allowed to drain freely, so nothing should be inserted in the nose. A nasogastric tube is avoided unless absolutely necessary because it may be inserted through the fracture into the brain. Clear fluid can be tested for glucose content using reagent strips; CSF usually tests positive, whereas mucus does not.

41. **(B)** The loss of consciousness that occurs with cerebral concussion usually is short, often only a few minutes. The alteration in consciousness clears spontaneously in 6–12 hours. The person usually has no memory of events just before the injury (retrograde amnesia) or just after it (anterograde amnesia). Post-concussion syndrome, manifested by persistent headache, confusion, and irritability, is a common sequela of concussion.

42. **(C)** This clinical situation fits the classic picture of epidural hematoma: a brief period of unconsciousness followed by a lucid interval, followed by a deteriorating level of consciousness. The patient's drowsiness should be reported promptly to the physician.

47. In the patient described in question 46, reflex activity may be expected to return following spinal shock. Reflex return could be assessed best by testing which of the following reflexes?

    A. Oculovestibular.
    B. Bulbocavernosus.
    C. Corneal.
    D. Biceps.

48. Which of the following is an expected finding during the early post-injury period in a person with a complete transection of the spinal cord above T_5?

    A. A pulse of 130.
    B. A blood pressure of 80/60.
    C. An intracranial pressure of 20 mm Hg.
    D. A vital capacity of 25 ml/kg.

49. A patient with a diagnosis of temporal lobe seizures would:

    A. Be expected to have sudden brief loss of muscle tone ("drop attacks").
    B. Be classified as having partial seizures with elemental symptomatology.
    C. Be likely to manifest amnesia following repetitive inappropriate activity.
    D. Display focal motor activity progressing up an extremity.

50. Which of the following is a pathophysiologic event occurring during status epilepticus?

    A. Hypothermia.
    B. Accumulation of high-energy phosphates.
    C. Cellular dehydration.
    D. Increased glycolysis.

Answers to Questions from page 76

43. (**B**) Chronic alcoholics are particularly difficult to evaluate owing to inebriation and progressive mental deterioration. In addition, they fall frequently because of alcohol's effects on cerebellar function. Finally, owing both to malnourishment and to impaired liver function, production of clotting factors is impaired. For these reasons, the alcoholic is at increased risk for an undetected chronic subdural hematoma.

44. (**D**) Bleeding into the brain parenchyma may result from rupture of an intracranial aneurysm, vessel rupture secondary to hypertension, arteriovenous malformations, trauma, or tumors. A fracture lacerating the middle meningeal artery would produce an epidural rather than intracerebral hematoma.

51. Of the following causes of status epilepticus, the most common is:

    A. Failure to take prescribed anticonvulsants.
    B. Acute alcohol withdrawal.
    C. Meningitis.
    D. Acute sedative withdrawal.

52. A continuously convulsing patient with an unknown history is brought to the critical care area of an emergency department. Which of the following drugs is most likely to be administered initially?

    A. Glucose.
    B. Naloxone.
    C. Sodium bicarbonate.
    D. Edrophonium chloride.

53. A patient develops status epilepticus because of failure to take prescribed anticonvulsants. In this situation, the initial anticonvulsant with route of choice for treatment of status epilepticus is:

    A. Intravenous diazepam.
    B. Oral phenobarbital.
    C. Intramuscular phenytoin.
    D. Oral paraldehyde.

54. When administering both diazepam and phenobarbital to control continuous seizures, the nurse should be aware of the potential for:

    A. Hyperexcitability.
    B. Hypoglycemia.
    C. Respiratory depression.
    D. Tachydysrhythmias.

55. Most intracranial (berry) aneurysms occur in the:

    A. Middle meningeal artery.
    B. Anterior vessels of the circle of Willis.
    C. Basilar artery.
    D. External carotid arteries.

56. A hypertensive patient complains of a sudden severe headache. She is at greatest risk for:

    A. Onset of migraine headaches.
    B. Vasovagal syncope due to pain.
    C. Ruptured intracranial aneurysm.
    D. Epidural hematoma.

45. **(D)** The injuries described are consistent with hemitransection of the cord (Brown-Séquard syndome). Pain and temperature sensations enter the cord via posterior roots and cross to the opposite side of the cord before ascending the spinothalamic tracts, so interruption of the tract causes loss of these sensations below the level of the lesion of the opposite side of the body. Motor (corticospinal) tracts cross in the medulla and descend on the same side of the cord as the muscles they innervate, so the cord injury causes same-sided paralysis.

    A total transection causes complete loss of sensory and voluntary motor function below the level of the lesion, because all sensory and motor spinal cord tracts are disrupted. An anterior cord syndrome produces (1) loss of pain and temperature sensation below the level of the lesion, because these sensations ascend the spinothalamic tracts in the anterolateral cord, (2) preservation of touch, vibration, and proprioception, because these sensations ascend the dorsal columns in the posterior cord, and (3) complete motor loss below the level of the lesion, because the corticospinal tracts are interrupted. (In addition, the anterior cord alone could not be injured by a stab wound to the back, the clinical presentation of this question.) A central cord syndrome results in varying sensory loss and greater weakness of the arms than of the legs, because the tracts to the cervical nerve roots are located near the center of the cord, and those to the sacral roots near the periphery.

46. **(B)** Injury at C_6 usually allows retention of gross arm movements (reaching forward) but not of intrinsic hand muscles, so fine coordination of fingers (picking up objects) is not possible. Diaphragmatic breathing is maintained with lesions below C_4. Because innervation to most chest muscles and all abdominal muscles is lost, the person needs support to sit upright.

57. A woman is hysterical following the abrupt death of her husband from a ruptured aneurysm. She sobs, "Why didn't he come to the hospital in time?" In comforting her, it would be most helpful to:

    A. Point out that aneurysm patients usually are well until the rupture occurs.
    B. Emphasize that what's done is done and there's no point in dwelling upon what cannot be changed.
    C. State that aneurysm patients are notorious for denial of symptoms.
    D. Say nothing because she won't be able to hear you anyway in her hysterical state.

58. A critical care nurse hears during shift report that a patient has been diagnosed as having a grade III aneurysm. The nurse realizes that the patient is:

    A. Awake with a minimal neurologic deficit.
    B. Lethargic with nuchal rigidity.
    C. Unresponsive and hemiplegic.
    D. Comatose and moribund.

59. A patient with a CVA of the left cerebral hemisphere would be likely to display all of the following manifestations *except*:

    A. Right hemiplegia.
    B. Right homonymous hemianopia.
    C. Aphasia.
    D. Deviation of eyes to the right.

Answers to Questions from page 78

47. (**B**) Spinal shock is a state of transient reflex depression below the level of the lesion, so testing the oculovestibular and corneal reflexes would not provide any information about reflex return. A patient with a C_6 injury would be expected to regain a biceps reflex. However, because reflexes tend to return in a rostral direction, with the bulbocavernosus reflex returning early, it would be most appropriate to evaluate reflex return by assessing the bulbocavernosus reflex. It can be checked by inserting a finger into the anus and feeling for contraction of the anal sphincter.

48. (**B**) In the early post-injury period (spinal shock), spinal cord injuries above T_5 usually produce a low blood pressure secondary to vasodilatation from loss of sympathetic stimulation from the transected cord. Rather than tachycardia, the person is likely to display bradycardia, again secondary to loss of sympathetic stimulation. An intracranial pressure of 20 mm Hg definitely is abnormal and merits prompt nursing action. Vital capacity is decreased rather than increased.

49. (**C**) Temporal lobe seizures most often manifest as automatisms, that is, repetitive nonpurposeful behaviors, such as smacking the lips and grimacing. The seizures are followed by amnesia for the seizure events. They are classified as partial seizures with complex symptomatology. Drop attacks are a type of generalized seizures. Focal motor activity progressing up an extremity, commonly called a jacksonian seizure, is a type of partial seizure with elemental symptomatology.

50. (**D**) Seizures are characterized by a marked increase in cerebral activity. Glycolysis increases to meet the accelerated demand for glucose. High-energy phosphates are depleted. Hyperthermia results from metabolic hyperactivity. Owing to the osmotic effects of increased intracellular byproducts of metabolism and to failure of the sodium-potassium pump, cellular swelling may occur.

60. When caring for a post-endarterectomy patient, the critical care nurse would be alert for all of the following operative-related complications *except*:

A. Excessive edema of the neck.
B. Ptosis of the eyelid.
C. Scalp ischemia.
D. Deviation of the tongue.

61. All of the following findings are consistent with meningeal irritation *except*:

A. Nuchal rigidity.
B. Headache.
C. Presence of Kernig's sign.
D. Presence of Trousseau's sign.

62. When caring for a person with meningitis, the critical care nurse should be alert for the development of which complication?

A. Cerebral dehydration.
B. Deafness.
C. Hypervigilance.
D. Hypothermia.

63. Which of the following statements correctly describes Guillain-Barré syndrome?

A. Paralysis occurs without prodromal symptoms.
B. The pathophysiologic process is irreversible.
C. The disease classically results in a descending paralysis.
D. Saltatory conduction is interrupted owing to demyelination of nerves.

Answers to Questions from page 79

51. (A) Although all the conditions mentioned can cause status epilepticus, the most common of them is interruption of prescribed anticonvulsant therapy.

52. (A) Given the clinical setting, the nurse should be prepared to administer glucose initially on the physician's orders. Glucose is indicated because hypoglycemia may precipitate seizures or may result from increased glucose consumption during prolonged seizure activity. Sodium bicarbonate may be necessary later to counteract the metabolic acidosis resulting from excessive metabolic activity. Naloxone is used to treat narcotic intoxication, whereas edrophonium chloride is used in the diagnosis of myasthenia gravis.

53. (A) Intravenous diazepam's onset of action is nearly immediate, making it the initial anticonvulsant of choice in this situation. Oral phenobarbital acts too slowly in this situation, intramuscular phenytoin is contraindicated because of its basic pH, and paraldehyde is administered only intravenously or intramuscularly in this setting because any oral medication would be inappropriate for a convulsing patient.

54. (C) Both diazepam and phenobarbital can cause respiratory depression, so the nurse should be particularly alert to this complication if both drugs are prescribed.

55. (B) Intracranial (berry) aneurysms usually arise at bifurcations of the arteries forming the circle of Willis. Typically, the anterior portion of the circle is involved. The remaining answers are all vessels outside the circle of Willis.

56. (C) Hypertension is a major contributing factor to rupture of an intracranial aneurysm. A migraine headache is a vascular phenomenon (arterial spasm followed by vasodilatation) but not particularly associated with hypertension. An epidural hematoma most often results from trauma. Vasovagal syncope (loss of consciousness due to massive parasympathetic discharge provoked by pain) is an unlikely occurrence given this clinical situation.

64. A patient with the Guillain-Barré syndrome might be expected to have which of the following complications?

    A. Autonomic dysfunction.
    B. Marked sensory loss.
    C. Diarrhea.
    D. Excessive bleeding.

65. Typical signs and symptoms reported by a person with generalized myasthenia gravis include:

    A. Early morning fatigability.
    B. Pain worsening with position changes.
    C. Weakness after sustained activity.
    D. Fecal incontinence.

66. The drug usually used to differentiate myasthenic from cholinergic crisis is:

    A. Edrophonium chloride (Tensilon).
    B. Phenytoin (Dilantin).
    C. Dopamine (Levodopa).
    D. Epinephrine (Adrenalin).

67. Three days after thymectomy, a patient is found crying about her operation. In responding to her, the nurse should be aware that:

    A. There is a variable lag time before the onset of remission after thymectomy.
    B. Symptoms persisting beyond 48 hours after operation indicate probable failure of the operative procedure.
    C. The patient probably is suffering from ICU psychosis.
    D. The stress manifested by crying can trigger a cholinergic crisis.

Answers to Questions from page 80

57. (**A**) In adjusting to the shock of a sudden death, family members often search for meaning for the death. Comforting but reality-based responses may help them to put the death in perspective. The first answer is both true and responsive to the person's question. The second answer, although true, could be perceived by the person as uncaring and cold. The third answer is untrue. The fourth is both untrue and unresponsive to the person's cry for help in understanding death.

58. (**B**) The most commonly used grading system has 5 categories. Categorization is useful in predicting the patient's need for nursing care as well as anticipating the treatment the physician may order and the outcome. The descriptions given as possible answers in A, B, C, and D are those of grades II, III, IV, and V, respectively. With grade I aneurysm, not mentioned in the question, the patient is alert with no neurologic deficit.

59. (**D**) As a general rule, the left cerebral hemisphere controls the right side of the body. When the left cerebral hemisphere is injured, the right side is paralyzed. In addition, since the left hemisphere is dominant for speech in most people, aphasia occurs. Loss of vision in the *right* half of *both* visual fields (right homonymous hemianopia) occurs because crossing of visual fibers at the optic chiasm causes visual impulses to be transmitted along the left optic tract and optic radiation to the left occipital lobe. The eyes will deviate to the left (where they can visualize) rather than the right.

68. Violent behavior is particularly characteristic of overdose of which type of drug?

    A. Barbiturate.
    B. Disulfiram.
    C. Phencyclidine.
    D. Acetaminophen.

69. Which of the following arterial blood gas findings is consistent with a diagnosis of salicylate poisoning?

    A. Respiratory and metabolic acidosis.
    B. Respiratory and metabolic alkalosis.
    C. Respiratory acidosis and metabolic alkalosis (with decreased anion gap).
    D. Respiratory alkalosis and metabolic acidosis (with increased anion gap).

70. Which of the following is a common complication of heroin overdose?

    A. Hepatic necrosis.
    B. Skin vesicles.
    C. Rhabdomyolysis.
    D. Non-cardiogenic pulmonary edema.

71. A primary danger of tricyclic antidepressant overdose is:

    A. Dysrhythmias.
    B. Renal failure.
    C. Gastrointestinal hemorrhage.
    D. Hypertensive crisis.

Answers to Questions from page 81

60. (**C**) Scalp ischemia is a complication of bypass grafts from extracranial to intracranial vessels rather than of endarterectomy. Edema around the operative site on the neck can compromise airway patency. Ptosis of the eyelid, often accompanied by pupil constriction and lack of sweating on the surgical side (Horner's syndrome), results from damage to sympathetic nerve fibers. The operative site is close to several cranial nerves. Deviation of the tongue indicates damage to the hypoglossal nerve. Damage to the other nerve most often affected, the vagus, results in vocal cord paralysis.

61. (**D**) Nuchal rigidity and headache are classic signs of meningeal irritation. Kernig's sign, which indicates meningitis, is elicited with the patient supine. The examiner flexes the patient's hip and knee and then straightens the knee. Pain or resistance on knee straightening (Kernig's sign) suggests meningeal irritation. Trousseau's sign, carpopedal spasms when an arm tourniquet is inflated, is present in hypocalcemia.

62. (**B**) Persistent neurologic deficits may occur with meningitis. If the 8th cranial nerve is involved, deafness may ensue. Cerebral edema occurs rather than dehydration, and hyperthermia rather than hypothermia. Hypervigilance is a sign found in selected psychiatric disorders.

63. (**D**) Saltatory conduction is conduction of nerve impulses along nodes of Ranvier (periodic interruptions of myelination). The Guillain-Barré syndrome is a disorder resulting from demyelination of nerves due to inflammation. With the loss of the myelin sheath, saltatory conduction is lost, making impulses travel more slowly down the nerve fibers. Paresthesias usually precede paralysis, which typically is an ascending paralysis. The disorder usually is reversible, with nerve function returning as remyelination occurs.

72. A patient with respiratory depression is brought to the critical care area of an emergency department after ingesting an unknown quantity of barbiturates. The nurse should anticipate a physician's order to first:

    A. Administer ipecac.
    B. Administer N-acetylcysteine.
    C. Assist with endotracheal intubation.
    D. Insert an Ewald tube.

73. A patient recovering from anesthesia would exhibit return of which function first?

    A. Swallowing reflex.
    B. Consciousness.
    C. Vomiting reflex.
    D. Cough reflex.

Answers to Questions from page 82

64. (**A**) The nurse should be alert for the development of autonomic dysfunction (most often manifested by marked fluctuations in blood pressure and pulse). Sensory loss, when present, is usually minimal; some patients instead experience hyperesthesia. GI dysfunction usually appears as gastric dilatation or ileus rather than diarrhea. Venous thrombosis and pulmonary embolus are more likely than excessive bleeding, because of immobility.

65. (**C**) The classic finding in myasthenia gravis is rapid weakness on exertion. Fatigue worsens as the day progresses. Pain is an uncommon finding, and poor bowel control is rare.

66. (**A**) Edrophonium chloride is a short-acting anticholinesterase utilized in the classic diagnostic test for myasthenia gravis and in differentiation of myasthenic from cholinergic crises. The symptoms will improve if the person is in myasthenic crisis and will worsen if the person is in cholinergic crisis.

67. (**A**) There is often a time lag of several months or years before a remission occurs after thymectomy. Because many patients perceive the operation as an "instant cure," continuing postoperative symptoms can be very disconcerting. The stress exhibited by the patient is unlikely to precipitate a cholinergic crisis (due to overdose of anticholinesterase drugs). Stress is more likely to trigger a myasthenic crisis. A cholinergic crisis, if one occurs, is more likely to result from increased sensitivity to anticholinesterases after thymectomy, which is an improvement in the disease process.

74. Reversal of neuromuscular blockade may be gauged by evaluating any of the following *except*:

    A. Hand grips.
    B. Tongue protrusion.
    C. Vital capacity.
    D. Cardiac rhythm.

75. If naloxone (Narcan) is given to reverse opiate depression, the nurse should be aware that:

    A. The usual dose is 8 mg IV bolus.
    B. Respiratory depression may later occur.
    C. Agitation following reversal is rare.
    D. The patient should first be intubated.

Answers to Questions from page 83

68. **(C)** Phencyclidine (PCP) is a psychedelic especially associated with violent behavior owing to its tendency to cause delusions. Barbiturate overdose usually causes a depressed level of consciousness. Disulfiram (Antabuse), a drug used by alcoholics to promote alcohol abstinence, causes a toxic reaction if the person ingests alcohol. Mild to moderate reactions involve throbbing headache, nausea and vomiting, confusion, and other symptoms, whereas severe reactions include respiratory depression and cardiovascular collapse. Acetaminophen overdose is marked by hepatotoxicity rather than changes in level of consciousness or behavior.

69. **(D)** Respiratory alkalosis results from hyperventilation because of direct stimulation of the respiratory center by salicylates. Metabolic acidosis with an increased anion gap results from the excess load of organic acids, which accumulates because of salicylate-induced changes in carbohydrate metabolism.

70. **(D)** Non-cardiogenic pulmonary edema occurs in $\frac{1}{4}$ to $\frac{1}{3}$ of patients suffering from acute heroin overdose. It may develop up to 24 hours after recovery of consciousness. Possible mechanisms are pulmonary capillary injury due to damage from adulterants used to "cut" the drug on the street; hypoxia; and anaphylaxis. Hepatic necrosis may occur with acetaminophen overdose. Skin vesicles are a sign of barbiturate overdose ("barb blisters"). Rhabdomyolysis (striated muscle destruction) may occur from the intense muscular effort exerted by a patient with PCP or other psychedelic intoxication.

71. **(A)** Tricyclic antidepressants have a marked impact on the cardiovascular system. Their cardiac effects are related to their anticholinergic activity and quinidine-like effects. They cause slowing of myocardial conduction, manifested particularly by widening of the QRS. A number of other electrocardiographic abnormalities and dysrhythmias also may be seen. Tricyclic overdoses also may produce significant hypotension owing to peripheral alpha-adrenergic blockage, which leads to vasodilatation.

Answers to Questions from page 84

72. **(C)** Induction of vomiting via ipecac administration is contraindicated in a person whose ability to protect the airway from aspiration is impaired. For the same reason, the person should undergo endotracheal intubation prior to passage of an Ewald tube. N-acetylcysteine is used in the treatment of acetaminophen overdose.

73. **(D)** The cough reflex returns first, followed by swallowing and vomiting reflexes. Consciousness returns last.

Answers to Questions from page 85

74. **(D)** Hand grips, tongue protrusion, and vital capacity are measures of muscular strength. Cardiac rhythm (an electrochemical event) is independent of muscular strength.

75. **(B)** Naloxone is a narcotic antagonist whose duration of action is shorter than that of narcotics. The patient should be observed closely for return of decreased level of consciousness and respiratory depression. Agitation is common on reversal of narcotic effect. The usual dose of naloxone is 0.4–0.8 mg IV bolus. Intubation prior to naloxone administration is unnecessary.

Bibliography

American Association of Critical-care Nurses. Core Curriculum for Critical Care Nursing, 3rd ed. W. B. Saunders, Philadelphia, 1985.
Current version of the classic outline of essential information for critical care nurses. Presented in a body systems format. Utilizes the four-step nursing process. Includes diagrams helpful in understanding complex concepts.

Auerbach, P., and Budassi, S. (eds.): Cardiac Arrest and CPR, 2nd ed. Aspen Systems Corp., Rockville, MD, 1983.
Although oriented primarily toward cardiovascular topics, this book contains useful discussions of the mechanisms of cerebral ischemia and postanoxic encephalopathy as well as barbiturate therapy following cardiac arrest.

Cosgriff, J., and Anderson, D.: The Practice of Emergency Care, 2nd ed. J. B. Lippincott Co., Philadelphia, 1984.
Excellent comprehensive reference on all types of emergencies. Salient anatomy, physiology, and pathophysiology presented succinctly. Numerous tables, charts, and diagrams emphasize key findings and interventions.

Cowley, R., and Trump, B. (eds.): Pathophysiology of Shock, Anoxia, and Ischemia. Williams & Wilkins Co., Baltimore, 1983.
Detailed, advanced-level content on pathophysiology of shock, anoxia, and ischemia. Several chapters contain in-depth discussions of interest to neuroscience nurses.

Greenbaum, D. M. (ed.): Clinical aspects of drug intoxication: the St. Vincent's Hospital Symposium. Heart Lung *12*(2 and 3), 1983.
Valuable collection of articles on recognition and clinical management of drug intoxication in the critical care unit as well as the emergency department. Articles included focus on general recognition and management; opioids and opiates; barbiturates, other sedatives, hypnotics, and tranquilizers; alcohol and miscellaneous agents; salicylates and acetaminophen; and tricyclic antidepressants.

Holloway, N.: Nursing the Critically Ill Adult: Applying Nursing Diagnosis, 2nd ed. Addison-Wesley Publishing Co., Menlo Park, CA, 1984.
Unique critical care text that uses nursing diagnosis framework for integration of anatomy and physiology, assessment, pathophysiology of common medical disorders, and nursing interventions. Appendices on legal issues in critical care, stress, and critical care pharmacology.

Kenner, C., Guzzetta, C., and Dossey, B. (eds.): Critical Care Nursing: Body-Mind-Spirit. Little, Brown and Co., Boston, 1981.
A beautifully presented work emphasizing the spiritual as well as the physiologic and psychological aspects of critical care nursing. Contains unique reflections on the art of critical care nursing.

Kinney, M., Dear, C., Packa, D., and Voorman, D. (eds.): AACN'S Clinical Reference for Critical-Care Nursing. McGraw-Hill Book Co., New York, 1981.
A comprehensive reference with a body systems approach. Both neuroanatomy and physiology chapter (by M. Ricci) and neurologic disorders chapter (by P. Mitchell) are clearly and concisely presented.

Nikas, D. (ed.): The Critically Ill Neurosurgical Patient. Churchill Livingstone, Inc., New York, 1982.
An advanced book focusing on concepts of importance in neurosurgical nursing. Contains detailed information on common topics, e.g., intracranial hypertension, as well as information difficult to find elsewhere, e.g., associations between neurologic disorders and cardiovascular disease.

Plum, F., and Posner, J.: The Diagnosis of Stupor and Coma, 3rd ed. F. A. Davis Co., Philadelphia, 1982.
A classic, highly detailed work focusing on the diagnosis of states of impaired consciousness. Contains many case presentations correlating signs and symptoms with findings on diagnostic procedures and autopsy. A fascinating reference most suitable to the experienced clinician, because content and discussion are on an advanced level.

Rudy, E.: Advanced Neurological and Neurosurgical Nursing. C. V. Mosby Co., St. Louis, 1984.
A detailed, easy-to-read presentation of neurologic and neurosurgical information on an advanced level. Useful both as introductory text for critical care nurses and as reference for experienced clinicians.

4 □ THE RENAL SYSTEM

CHAROLD L. BAER

1. An individual with fewer juxtamedullary nephrons than normal would have a decreased capacity for implementing which of the following processes?

    A. Excreting waste products.
    B. Concentrating urine.
    C. Filtering blood.
    D. Reabsorbing electrolytes.

2. Damage to the basement membrane of the glomerulus would result in production of a filtrate containing abnormal amounts of which of the following substances?

    A. Protein and sodium.
    B. Glucose and white blood cells.
    C. Urea and creatinine.
    D. Albumin and red blood cells.

3. Given the following pressure values in relation to the glomerulus and Bowman's capsule—an intracapsular pressure of 10 mm Hg; a serum colloid osmotic pressure of 30 mm Hg; and an intracapillary hydrostatic pressure of 60 mm Hg—what is the net filtration pressure?

    A. 20 mm Hg.
    B. 40 mm Hg
    C. 80 mm Hg.
    D. 100 mm Hg.

4. A patient who is voiding 20 ml per hour has the following lab values:

	Serum	Urine
Sodium	146 mEq/L	14 mEq/L
Potassium	5.8 mEq/L	20 mEq/L
Chloride	106 mEq/L	30 mEq/L
BUN	60 mg	—
Creatinine	4 mg/100 ml	900 mg/100 ml
Osmolality	—	450 mOsm/kg H_2O

What is the patient's creatinine clearance (Ccr) or glomerular filtration rate (GFR)?

    A. 45 ml/min.
    B. 68 ml/min.
    C. 75 ml/min.
    D. 125 ml/min.

5. Which of the following concepts accurately describes the process that occurs when a substance such as glucose, which is normally not present in the urine, suddenly appears in the urine?

   A. Saturated passive diffusion gradient.
   B. Diminished active ion transport.
   C. Maximal transport capacity.
   D. Maximal clearance capacity.

6. A patient with a serum osmolality of 310 mOsm/L, who has an adequately functioning ADH-osmoreceptor mechanism, would exhibit which of the following urine specific gravities?

   A. 1.003.
   B. 1.010.
   C. 1.015.
   D. 1.030.

7. The countercurrent mechanism of the kidney is dependent on which of the following factors?

   A. A hairpin structure and a sodium chloride pump.
   B. A hypertonic medullary interstitium and ADH.
   C. Urea back-diffusion and aldosterone.
   D. The vasa recta and cortical glomeruli.

8. A patient with dysfunctional proximal tubules is likely to experience which of the following sets of electrolyte imbalances?

   A. Hyperchloremia and hyperkalemia.
   B. Hypokalemia and hypocalcemia.
   C. Hypernatremia and hypochloremia.
   D. Hyponatremia and hypercalcemia.

9. Which of the following sets of fluid and electrolyte imbalances would you expect to find in a patient who is secreting abnormally high amounts of aldosterone?

   A. Hypernatremia and hypokalemia.
   B. Hypervolemia and hyponatremia.
   C. Hyperkalemia and hypovolemia.
   D. Hyperkalemia and hypernatremia.

10. Which of the following is a likely result of increased parathyroid hormone (PTH) secretion?

    A. Decreased hydroxylation of vitamin D.
    B. Increased tubular reabsorption of calcium.
    C. Decreased tubular excretion of phosphate.
    D. Increased mineralization of the bones.

11. In a patient experiencing metabolic acidosis, which of the following electrolyte imbalances is likely to be present?

    A. Hypocalcemia.
    B. Hyponatremia.
    C. Hyperkalemia.
    D. Hyperphosphatemia.

Answers to Questions from page 89

1. (**B**) The juxtamedullary nephrons have long loops of Henle, which penetrate deeply into the medulla. These long loops participate in the countercurrent multiplication and exchange mechanism that is responsible for concentrating and diluting the urine.

2. (**D**) The glomerular basement membrane is normally impermeable to large protein molecules, albumin, red blood cells, and white blood cells. It is permeable to all of the other substances listed.

3. (**A**) Net filtration pressure is the difference between those pressures that facilitate filtration and those that oppose it. Intracapillary hydrostatic pressure supports filtration, whereas intracapsular and colloid osmotic pressures oppose it. Thus, 60 mm Hg minus 40 mm Hg equals the net filtration pressure.

4. (**C**) The formula used in determining the clearance of a substance is identical to the formula used to calculate glomerular filtration rate:

$$\text{GFR or Ccr} = \frac{(U_{cr} \times V)}{P_{cr}}$$

where cr = creatinine; U_{cr} = the urine concentration of creatinine; V = the flow rate of urine per minute; and P_{cr} = the plasma concentration of creatinine.

12. In which of the following patients, none of whom has renal failure, would you expect to see an elevated BUN?

   A. The patient receiving an 80 gm protein diet.
   B. The septic patient.
   C. The hypervolemic patient.
   D. The stable patient one day after an operation.

13. Which of the following pairs of conditions best describes the urine excreted by most patients experiencing chronic renal dysfunction?

   A. Hypernaturia and hypertonicity.
   B. Hypertonicity and glycosuria.
   C. Hypokaluria and isotonicity.
   D. Hypercalciuria and hypotonicity.

14. The skin of a patient experiencing renal dysfunction is best described by which of the following sets of three adjectives?

   A. Pale, oily, and abraded.
   B. Pink, abraded, and wrinkled.
   C. Yellow, dry, and bruised.
   D. Cyanotic, edematous, and dry.

15. A renal dysfunction patient receiving which of the following medications would be at risk for developing tetany?

   A. Aluminum hydroxide.
   B. 1,25-Dihydroxycholecalciferol.
   C. Intravenous furosemide.
   D. Intravenous sodium bicarbonate.

16. Which of the following sets of vital signs most accurately represents those of a patient experiencing renal dysfunction?

   A. BP 132/88; P 84; R 16; T 98.6.
   B. BP 140/90; P 90; R 20; T 100.6.
   C. BP 160/96; P 100; R 32; T 99.
   D. BP 170/102; P 132; R 28; T 102.

17. Which of the following sets of imbalances occurs in the serum of a patient experiencing renal dysfunction?

   A. Uremia, hyperchloremia, and hypercalcemia.
   B. Hyperkalemia, hypocalcemia, and hyperphosphatemia.
   C. Hypernatremia, hypokalemia, and uremia.
   D. Hyponatremia, hypochloremia, and hypophosphatemia.

Answers to Questions from page 90

5. (**C**) The tubules have maximal capacities for reabsorbing and secreting substances. When the specific tubular transport capacity for a given substance is surpassed, the substance will appear in either the urine or the blood in abnormal amounts. The amount of the substance in either the urine or the blood depends on whether it is normally reabsorbed or secreted. If it is normally reabsorbed, it will now appear in increased amounts in the urine; if it is normally secreted, it will now appear in increased amounts in the blood.

6. (**D**) A serum osmolality of 310 mOsm/L would trigger the ADH-osmoreceptor mechanism, and increased amounts of ADH would be secreted. In response to the increased secretion of ADH, the distal tubules and collecting ducts would reabsorb more water. The result would be a very hypertonic urine.

7. (**A**) The countercurrent mechanism functions to concentrate urine. It is able to perform this function because of the hairpin structure of the long loops of Henle and the interactions between that structure, a hypertonic medullary interstitium, and the vasa recta. The medullary interstitium acts as a reservoir from which sodium and chloride are pumped into the curve of the loop of Henle to increase the osmolality of the filtrate. The vasa recta serve to maintain the solute load in the medullary interstitium in order to maintain the reservoir. Urea back-diffusion assists in generating and maintaining a hypertonic medullary interstitium.

8. (**B**) The proximal tubule is the active reabsorption site for 65% of the filtered sodium and calcium. It is also the major site for active potassium reabsorption and passive chloride reabsorption. Dysfunctional proximal tubules would result in decreased reabsorption of those ions and thus create lower levels in the blood.

9. (**A**) Aldosterone acts in the distal tubule to augment sodium reabsorption in exchange for potassium and hydrogen ion secretion. Thus, increased aldosterone secretion results in hypervolemia, hypernatremia, hypokalemia, and metabolic alkalosis.

18. Which of the following creatinine clearance values would be consistent with a diagnosis of actual, intrinsic renal failure?

    A. 5 ml/min.
    B. 20 ml/min.
    C. 80 ml/min
    D. 100 ml/min.

19. Which of the following assessment data are consistent with hypovolemia?

    A. Increased pulse and a swollen tongue.
    B. Neck vein distention and dry skin.
    C. Weight loss and thirst.
    D. Increased blood pressure and a fever.

20. You would be most concerned about decreased nutritional intake in a patient with renal dysfunction because it might result in:

    A. Hypocalcemia.
    B. Hypoglycemia.
    C. Increased protein anabolism.
    D. Increased tissue catabolism.

21. Which of the following imbalances are frequently seen as a result of diuretic therapy?

    A. Hyperuricemia and hypokalemia.
    B. Hypernatremia and metabolic alkalosis.
    C. Hyperchloremia and metabolic acidosis.
    D. Hyponatremia and hyperkalemia.

22. A patient experiencing renal dysfunction suddenly complains of decreased auditory acuity. Which of the following medications is the probable cause of the deficit?

    A. Hydralazine.
    B. Propranolol.
    C. Furosemide.
    D. Folic acid.

23. Which of the following types of diuretics would be appropriately prescribed for a patient who requires an alkaline urine?

    A. An aldosterone inhibitor.
    B. A carbonic anhydrase inhibitor.
    C. A loop diuretic.
    D. An osmotic diuretic.

Answers to Questions from page 91

10. (**B**) An increase in parathyroid hormone secretion results in increases in distal tubular reabsorption of calcium, tubular excretion of phosphate, and hydroxylation of vitamin D as well as demineralization of the bones.

11. (**C**) In metabolic acidosis, potassium shifts extracellularly as hydrogen moves intracellularly, resulting in hyperkalemia.

24. Which of the following nursing interventions is appropriate when caring for an individual who is receiving a diuretic?

   A. Monitor blood pressures and give tomato juice.
   B. Monitor pulses and give bouillon.
   C. Monitor daily weights and give bananas.
   D. Monitor output and give potato chips.

25. Which of the following groups of medications are usually prescribed for a patient experiencing renal failure?

   A. Antianemics, antacids, and antihypertensives.
   B. Diuretics, multivitamins, and antidepressants.
   C. Cardiotonics, analgesics, and immunosuppressants.
   D. Cathartics, anticoagulants, and calcium preparations.

26. Which of the following antihypertensive agents often requires that a beta-blocker be given as adjunctive therapy?

   A. Captopril.
   B. Clonidine.
   C. Hydralazine.
   D. Methyldopa.

27. Which of the following sets of symptoms is characteristic of uremia?

   A. Nausea and seborrhea.
   B. Dementia and lethargy.
   C. Ascites and gastritis.
   D. Pruritus and stomatitis.

28. The best nursing intervention to use in minimizing uremia in a patient would be to:

   A. Restrict fluids.
   B. Restrict protein.
   C. Give sodium bicarbonate.
   D. Increase physical activity.

Answers to Questions from page 92

12. (**B**) The catabolic processes involved in sepsis will produce additional breakdown products of protein metabolism. Urea is one of these products, and increased amounts of it will elevate the BUN.

13. (**C**) The patient with chronic renal dysfunction has insufficient tubular function to secrete and excrete potassium ions or to concentrate or dilute urine. In addition, the normal tubular responses to all of the other electrolytes are also altered. The result is a relatively isotonic urine with significantly lower amounts of electrolytes than normal.

14. (**C**) In renal dysfunction, urochrome pigments are retained and deposited in the skin, producing a yellowish coloration. In addition, the oil glands do not function appropriately, so the skin is abnormally dry. Also, the alterations in clotting, as well as the capillary fragility produced by uremia, predispose the patient to easy bruising.

15. (**D**) When acidosis is rapidly corrected, there is a decrease in the amount of ionized calcium available. This decrease creates a depletion of calcium in the extracellular fluid and predisposes the patient to develop tetany.

16. (**C**) The patient with renal dysfunction would have increased blood pressure and pulse because of fluid overload and electrolyte imbalances. The patient's respirations would be increased to compensate for metabolic acidosis, and the body temperature would be relatively normal.

17. (**B**) The patient in renal dysfunction retains potassium and phosphate because the tubules cannot secrete or excrete those ions. The increase in serum phosphate depresses the serum calcium, which is then deposited in soft tissues.

29. You would expect a patient with renal dysfunction to exhibit which of the following sets of psychological responses as part of the coping process?

    A. Depression and denial.
    B. Dependency and delusions.
    C. Anxiety and hysteria.
    D. Regression and hallucinations.

30. In which phases of oliguric acute renal failure is the patient most susceptible to developing severe fluid and electrolyte imbalances?

    A. The onset and oliguric phases.
    B. The oliguric and early diuretic phases.
    C. The oliguric and late diuretic phases.
    D. The late diuretic and recovery phases.

31. The most appropriate nursing intervention to use in dealing with the deep, rapid respirations exhibited by a patient experiencing acute renal failure would be to:

    A. Elevate the head of the bed and administer sodium bicarbonate as prescribed.
    B. Turn the patient and institute coughing and deep breathing exercises every 2 hours.
    C. Promote rest and administer medications prescribed to decrease the respiratory rate.
    D. Position the patient upright in bed and administer oxygen at 5 L/min per nasal cannula.

32. The drowsiness and confusion that are often seen in patients experiencing acute renal failure are due to:

    A. Hypoxia.
    B. Metabolic acidosis.
    C. Hypernatremia.
    D. Hyperkalemia.

33. Which of the following sets of data is consistent with a diagnosis of prerenal oliguria?

    A. A urine sodium of 8 mEq/L and a urine specific gravity of 1.028.
    B. A urine sodium of 30 mEq/L and no proteinuria.
    C. A BUN of 40 mg and a serum creatinine of 5 mg.
    D. Tubular casts and a urine specific gravity of 1.020.

Answers to Questions from page 93

18. (**A**) The individual in renal failure would have a creatinine clearance of less than 5 ml/min. The other values could indicate hypoperfusion states or progressing renal insufficiency, but not failure.

19. (**C**) Fluid loss is rapidly manifested by decreases in body weight. Also, the increase in serum osmolality that occurs because of hypovolemia triggers the thirst center in the hypothalamus, engendering an increased desire to drink water.

20. (**D**) Decreased nutritional intake forces the body to utilize its own tissues as an energy source. This condition results in muscle wasting and an increase in the waste products of protein metabolism.

21. (**A**) Most diuretics work by inhibiting sodium and chloride reabsorption in the loop of Henle or the distal tubule. An increase in the amount of sodium delivered to the distal tubule facilitates the tubular exchange of sodium and potassium ions. Thus, large amounts of potassium are excreted as well. Also, many diuretics (particularly small doses of thiazides) promote the reabsorption of urates and predispose the patient to hyperuricemia.

22. (**C**) Furosemide has frequently been documented as producing transient deafness in patients through its toxic effect on the 8th cranial nerve. Fortunately, this is usually a reversible dysfunction.

23. (**B**) Diuretics that function by inhibiting carbonic anhydrase decrease the ability of the tubules to generate and secrete hydrogen ions. They also inhibit proximal tubular reabsorption of filtered bicarbonate. These effects cause the distal tubule to be flooded with more bicarbonate than it can effectively reabsorb, creating a loss of bicarbonate in the urine and producing an alkaline urine.

34. Which of the following sets of data is consistent with a diagnosis of oliguria resulting from gentamicin therapy?

    A. Tubular casts and no proteinuria.
    B. Heavy proteinuria and a urine sodium of 10 mEq/L.
    C. A urine specific gravity of 1.008 and a BUN of 30 mg.
    D. A urine sodium of 40 mEq/L and a urine specific gravity of 1.010.

35. Which of the following nursing interventions are appropriate for caring for a patient with newly diagnosed prerenal oliguria?

    A. Restrict fluids and prepare the patient for dialysis.
    B. Give fluids and prepare the patient for x-ray.
    C. Administer a fluid challenge and give diuretics as prescribed.
    D. Restrict fluids and give insulin and glucose as prescribed.

36. A patient in the diuretic phase of acute renal failure would benefit most from which of the following therapeutic interventions?

    A. Give fluids at 30 ml per hour.
    B. Give fluids at 30 ml plus the urine output per hour.
    C. Give fluids at 30 ml plus 2/3 of the urine output per hour.
    D. Give fluids at 25 ml per hour.

37. Which of the following nursing interventions would be appropriate for caring for a patient in the late diuretic phase of acute renal failure?

    A. Provide a diet high in calories and low in protein.
    B. Insert a Foley catheter.
    C. Initiate dialysis.
    D. Administer prophylactic antibiotics as prescribed.

Answers to Questions from page 94

24. (**C**) All of the monitoring functions are appropriate for caring for an individual receiving diuretics. However, the only food item of the four that are appropriate to be given is bananas, which will replace lost potassium. All of the other food items are high in sodium and/or fluid content and should not be given because they would counteract the effect of the diuretic.

25. (**A**) The patient experiencing renal failure is anemic, hyperphosphatemic, uremic, and hypertensive. These medications would be of benefit in treating those problems. All of the other medications would also be appropriate *except* for the antidepressants and, in many cases, the immunosuppressants and anticoagulants. In addition, only selected analgesics, cathartics, and antacids can be used with these patients. Aluminum-based antacids are preferred, and magnesium containing antacids are contraindicated.

26. (**C**) Hydralazine is a vasodilator that relaxes smooth muscle and decreases peripheral resistance. The sympathetic nervous system response to this action produces a reflex tachycardia that is counteracted by the beta blocker.

27. (**D**) The deposition of calcium-phosphate products in the skin, accompanied by the effects of uremic toxins on the nerve endings, produces pruritus in the uremic patient. The breakdown of urea produces ulcers not only in the mouth but also in the gastrointestinal mucosa. The effect of uremic toxins on the central nervous system produces the lethargy and some of the nausea in addition to other manifestations. Nausea is also an effect of the toxins on the gastrointestinal mucosa. Seborrhea, dementia, and ascites, however, are not usually directly attributable to uremia.

28. (**B**) Restricting protein intake decreases the nitrogenous metabolic waste products that would accumulate in the body and add to the uremic state.

38. A patient who is undergoing peritoneal dialysis experiences abdominal discomfort, and you note that the dialysate outflow for the 12th exchange is bloody. What is the most likely explanation for this change in the dialysate outflow?

   A. Peritonitis.
   B. Bowel perforation.
   C. Bladder perforation.
   D. Abdominal wall erosion.

39. A patient who is undergoing peritoneal dialysis using 2-liter exchanges of 4.25% solution with 8 mEq of KCl added is likely to develop which of the following sets of imbalances?

   A. Hypovolemia and hyperkalemia.
   B. Hypovolemia and hyperglycemia.
   C. Hyponatremia and hypokalemia.
   D. Hyponatremia and hyperchloremia.

40. Which of the following sets of signs and symptoms is manifested by patients with chronic renal failure?

   A. Anorexia, lassitude, and seborrhea.
   B. Muscle wasting, tinnitus, and gastritis.
   C. Yellow skin, decreased libido, and hypertension.
   D. Soft tissue calcifications, dysphagia, and fatigue.

41. Which of the following sets of data about a patient's urine would lead you to suspect that the patient had end stage renal disease?

   A. White cell casts and pyuria.
   B. Waxy casts and proteinuria.
   C. Hyaline casts and dysuria.
   D. Lymphocyte casts and eosinophiluria.

42. A patient experiencing chronic renal failure develops frank gastrointestinal bleeding. Which of the following reasons accurately explains your concern regarding this complication?

   A. It will make the patient more anorexic.
   B. It will make the patient more uremic.
   C. It will interfere with the absorption of nutrients.
   D. It will result in a loss of fluid and electrolytes.

Answers to Questions from page 95

29. (A) Depression, denial, dependency, and regression are all normal psychological responses that may be expressed in the process of coping with a chronic illness. The other responses are pathologic and signify mental dysfunction.

30. (C) The patient in acute renal failure is likely to experience wide variations in fluid and electrolyte balance during: (1) the oliguric phase, when minimal excretion results in fluid overload and excessive amounts of most electrolytes, and (2) the late diuretic phase, when the kidney begins to excrete not only large volumes of fluid but also large quantities of electrolytes.

31. (A) The patient in acute renal failure exhibits deep, rapid respirations as a compensatory mechanism to deal with the existing metabolic acidosis. This respiratory pattern should be supported, and additional measures should be implemented to treat the acidosis. Administering sodium bicarbonate would be one such measure.

32. (B) The metabolic acidosis that results from the inability of the tubules to secrete and excrete hydrogen ions acts as a depressant on the central nervous system. Those depressive effects are manifested in the patient as drowsiness, confusion, lethargy, weakness, and decreased mentation.

33. (A) In prerenal oliguria, there is a decrease in perfusion but no tubular damage. Thus, the tubules can still reabsorb sodium and concentrate urine. In fact, the tubules accomplish those functions quite well in an attempt to restore renal perfusion.

43. Which of the following is an infrequently seen manifestation of renal failure?

   A. Pulmonary edema.
   B. Metastatic calcifications.
   C. Pericardial effusion.
   D. Uremic frost.

44. A patient with chronic renal failure presents with the following signs and symptoms: hypotension, jugular vein distention, severe chest pain, distant heart sounds, and a rapid, weak pulse. The most appropriate nursing intervention to use in caring for this patient would be to:

   A. Initiate dialysis immediately.
   B. Administer nitroglycerin and digoxin as prescribed.
   C. Prepare the patient for a pericardiocentesis.
   D. Give intravenous fluids and obtain an ECG.

45. A patient with chronic renal failure presents with the following signs and symptoms: dyspnea, tachycardia, rales, frothy hemoptysis, an S_3 gallop, and hypotension. The most effective and efficient nursing intervention to use in caring for this patient would be to

   A. Initiate dialysis immediately.
   B. Elevate the head of the bed and give digoxin as prescribed.
   C. Administer oxygen and give diuretics as prescribed.
   D. Institute rotating tourniquets on the extremities.

46. Which of the following pairs of complications is a patient with chronic renal failure likely to develop?

   A. Angina and pleuritis.
   B. Jaundice and epistaxis.
   C. Paresthesias and foot drop.
   D. Asterixis and phlebitis.

47. The adult patient with chronic renal failure is likely to experience which of the following complications in relation to the endocrine system?

   A. Hypogonadism.
   B. Pancreatitis.
   C. Hypothyroidism.
   D. Hyperparathyroidism.

Answers to Questions from page 96

34. (**D**) Gentamicin is a nephrotoxic aminoglycoside that produces intrarenal acute renal failure by damaging renal tubules and producing acute tubular necrosis. Following severe tubular damage, reflex mechanisms in the kidney decrease the blood flow to the involved nephrons, thus decreasing GFR. The result is that the kidneys produce a urine with the same specific gravity as plasma (1.010). In addition, the tubules cannot reabsorb electrolytes as efficiently as they normally do, so sodium wasting occurs. Also, tubular casts and mild to moderate proteinuria are often seen.

35. (**C**) Newly diagnosed prerenal oliguria can be reversed before it progresses to intrarenal acute renal failure. Usually, therapeutic interventions must be initiated within 4 to 8 hours of the onset of the oliguria in order to be effective. Administering fluids and diuretics are two of the therapeutic interventions that can reverse the renal hypoperfusion created by prerenal etiologies.

36. (**C**) During the diuretic phase, it is important to replace fluids, including those lost through insensible mechanisms. However, it is essential that not all of the urine output be replaced in order to encourage the tubular concentration processes.

37. (**A**) The patient in the late diuretic phase of acute renal failure is excreting large volumes of fluids with varying solute loads. Thus, in order to minimize the uremic manifest .tions, a low-protein diet is required, and adequate calories must be provided to prevent tissue catabolism. All of the other interventions are inappropriate for a patient in the late diuretic phase of acute renal failure.

48. Which of the following nursing interventions are the most appropriate for dealing with the integumentary system of a patient with chronic renal failure?

    A. Bathe the patient q.o.d. and give Benadryl as prescribed.
    B. Bathe the patient daily and apply a lubricating oil.
    C. Cleanse the skin with soap and apply lanolin.
    D. Cleanse the skin with alcohol and give Temaril as prescribed.

49. Administration of which of the following substances is likely to assist in reversing the impotence experienced by chronic renal failure patients?

    A. Phosphate.
    B. Testosterone.
    C. Decadurabolin.
    D. Zinc.

50. Which of the following sets of antacids would be most appropriately prescribed for a patient experiencing chronic renal failure?

    A. Alternagel and Amphojel.
    B. Basaljel and Aludrox.
    C. Camalox and Maalox.
    D. Mylanta and Riopan.

51. During which of the following periods is the renal transplant patient at risk for developing accelerated rejection?

    A. 1 to 4 hours after operation.
    B. 2 to 5 days after operation.
    C. 1 to 3 weeks after operation.
    D. 6 to 12 months after operation.

52. Which of the following types of rejection are irreversible?

    A. Accelerated and acute.
    B. Hyperacute and acute.
    C. Accelerated and chronic.
    D. Hyperacute and chronic.

Answers to Questions from page 97

38. (**D**) The appearance of bloody dialysate outflow after the initial four to six exchanges usually indicates some type of trauma to the abdominal wall or viscera. Peritonitis can also occasionally produce blood-tinged dialysate; however, this sign is almost always accompanied by the other clinical manifestations of peritonitis. If the dialysate outflow was bloody after the 1st exchange and continued to be bloody throughout the remaining exchanges, uremic coagulopathy may be the cause.

39. (**B**) The hypertonic glucose solution will osmotically remove fluid. Also, as the solution remains in the abdominal cavity, some of the glucose will be absorbed, predisposing the patient to develop hyperglycemia.

40. (**C**) The patient with chronic renal failure manifests all of these signs and symptoms *except* for seborrhea, tinnitus, and dysphagia. None of those three latter symptoms is directly attributable to uremia. In general, the other signs and symptoms are a result of the effects of uremic toxins on various body systems, acid-base imbalances, and fluid and electrolyte imbalances.

41. (**B**) Proteinuria indicates damage to the glomerular membrane, and waxy casts are present only in end stage renal disease patients. The other data are characteristic of urinary tract infections, normal urine, or acute interstitial nephritis.

42. (**B**) Blood is protein, and when it is absorbed from the gastrointestinal system it must be metabolized. As it is metabolized, it increases the amount of protein breakdown products in the body and accentuates the uremic state.

53. A patient who has just received a renal transplant from a living relative returns to the unit from the recovery room. You notice that the patient's urine output is now only 60 ml per hour, although in the recovery room it had been 100–250 ml per hour. The patient complains of abdominal fullness, and you note some change in abdominal girth, but all vital signs remain stable. What is the most likely explanation for the change in the patient's state?

   A. Hyperacute rejection.
   B. A leaking renal artery anastomosis.
   C. A leaking ureterovesical anastomosis.
   D. Acute pancreatitis.

54. Which of the following immunosuppressant agents is the most specific for inhibiting cell-mediated immunity?

   A. Azathioprine.
   B. Cyclophosphamide.
   C. Cyclosporin A.
   D. Prednisone.

55. Which of the following are major side effects of long term corticosteroid therapy?

   A. Hyperglycemia and cataracts.
   B. Anorexia and edema.
   C. Alopecia and anemia.
   D. Jaundice and acne.

56. A 24-year-old male college student is admitted to the hospital following a hard tackle in a football game. He is semicomatose and there is a large hematoma over his right flank. He has hematuria, a urine output of 70 ml per hour, and a urine specific gravity of 1.026. He currently has an I.V. of D5/.45 NS infusing at 100 ml per hour. What is the probable cause of this patient's hematuria?

   A. A renal contusion.
   B. A renal laceration.
   C. A renal fracture.
   D. A renal pedicle disruption.

Answers to Questions from page 98

43. (**D**) The presence of urea crystals on the skin as uremic frost is a relatively infrequent manifestation of renal dysfunction. Most patients who develop this manifestation are inadequately dialyzed and may have poor hygienic habits.

44. (**C**) The patient is exhibiting the classic signs and symptoms of cardiac tamponade, and a pericardiocentesis is mandatory to alleviate the problem.

45. (**A**) Dialysis therapy is the most effective and efficient method for removing the excess fluid to alleviate the complication of pulmonary edema and improve the cardiovascular status. The other interventions would be only adjunctive.

46. (**C**) The effect of uremic toxins on the nervous system results in a slowing of nerve conduction velocity and segmental demyelination of the nerves. The patient experiences peripheral neuropathy, which progresses from paresthesias to foot drop and, on rare occasions, even to paralysis. Uremic toxins may also produce asterixis and pleuritis. In addition, epistaxis may be seen in patients with uremic coagulopathy.

47. (**D**) Patients with chronic renal failure develop hyperphosphatemia owing to decreased renal excretion of phosphorus. Hyperphosphatemia results in a continuously depressed level of serum calcium, which produces secondary hyperparathyroidism. This latter state results from the hypersecretion of parathormone in response to the decreased extracellular calcium levels.

57. Which of the following pairs of findings would be consistent with a diagnosis of renal trauma accompanied by normal renal function?

    A. Hypovolemia and increased creatinine.
    B. Decreased hematocrit and hypocalcemia.
    C. Increased BUN and hyperkalemia.
    D. Hypokalemia and hypernatremia.

58. Which of the following conditions would require surgical intervention?

    A. A subcapsular hematoma.
    B. Urinary extravasation.
    C. A cortical laceration.
    D. A medullary laceration.

59. The most appropriate nursing interventions to use in caring for a patient newly diagnosed as having a renal contusion are to

    A. Force fluids and encourage ambulation.
    B. Monitor the urine for hematuria and prepare the patient for surgery.
    C. Encourage bedrest and administer analgesics as prescribed.
    D. Restrict fluids and administer antibiotics as prescribed.

60. Which of the following sets of signs and symptoms would be exhibited by a patient with a serum potassium of 6.8 mEq/L?

    A. Bradycardia and constipation.
    B. Confusion and muscle cramps.
    C. Paralytic ileus and paresthesias.
    D. Diarrhea and flaccid paralysis.

61. Which of the following therapeutic measures will reduce total body potassium levels?

    A. Calcium gluconate.
    B. Glucose and insulin.
    C. Kayexalate.
    D. Sodium bicarbonate.

62. A patient with a potassium of 2.2 mEq/L is at increased risk for developing which of the following complications?

    A. Bowel perforation.
    B. Hypertensive crisis.
    C. Seizures.
    D. Carpopedal spasms.

Answers to Questions from page 99

48. **(B)** It is important to cleanse the patient's skin at least daily in order to keep the pores open so they can act as organs of excretion for waste products. Applying oil or lotion helps maintain the integrity of the skin and assists in decreasing the pruritis. It is important that nonirritating, non-drying, non–lanolin-based substances be used in caring for the skin.

49. **(D)** The impotence may be partially due to a deficiency in zinc in the patient's diet. The androgenic substances will not assist in correcting impotence but may assist in treating the patient's anemia. Giving phosphates will increase the secretion of parathyroid hormone, only enhancing the impotence.

50. **(A)** Antacids are given to chronic renal failure patients not only to neutralize gastric acidity but also to bind phosphate so it can be excreted in the feces. Such antacids need to be low in magnesium and sodium in order not to produce additional electrolyte imbalances.

51. **(B)** Accelerated rejection is physiologically similar to a hyperacute rejection episode, and thus, it usually occurs in the first few postoperative days.

52. **(D)** Hyperacute rejection is an immunologic response to pre-existing antibodies that creates an irreversible ischemia by occluding small renal arteries. Chronic rejection is a slow immunologic response that involves deterioration of the glomerular basement membrane, tubular necrosis, and interstitial fibrosis. This type of rejection ultimately results in organ failure.

63. Which of the following nursing interventions are appropriate when caring for a patient who has a potassium of 2.9 mEq/L?

    A. Monitor respirations and give diuretics as prescribed.
    B. Monitor level of consciousness and give sodium bicarbonate as prescribed.
    C. Monitor intake and output and give raisins.
    D. Monitor bowel sounds and give cranberry juice.

64. The following serum laboratory values were obtained from a patient on your unit:

Na 152 mEq/L	Ca 12.0 mg/dl
K 5.0 mEq/L	PO_4 3.2 mg/dl
Cl 110 mEq/L	Mg 1.8 mEq/L

    Which electrolyte imbalances would you expect the patient to exhibit?

    A. Hypernatremia, hypophosphatemia, and hypomagnesemia.
    B. Hyperkalemia, hypophosphatemia, and hypercalcemia.
    C. Hyperchloremia, hypomagnesemia, and hypernatremia.
    D. Hypernatremia, hyperchloremia, and hypercalcemia.

65. Which of the following nursing interventions are appropriate in caring for a patient who is experiencing hypernatremia due to excessive water loss?

    A. Provide for oral hygiene and administer .45 NS I.V. as prescribed.
    B. Monitor weight and give tomato juice.
    C. Bathe with cool water and administer Ringer's lactate as prescribed.
    D. Monitor central nervous system status and give bouillon.

66. Which of the following conditions would account for a serum sodium of 128 mEq/L?

    A. Hyperaldosteronism.
    B. Hyperglycemia.
    C. Fever.
    D. Unconsciousness.

Answers to Questions from page 100

53. (**C**) A rapid change in urine output accompanied by abdominal fullness in the immediate postoperative period with no alteration in vital signs strongly indicates a leaking or incomplete ureterovesical anastomosis. Significant alterations in vital signs would suggest a leaking vascular anastomosis.

54. (**C**) Cyclosporin A produces almost total inhibition of T cells with relatively little effect on B cells. It also inhibits T helper cells but may spare T suppressor cells.

55. (**A**) Glucocorticoids promote gluconeogenesis by: (1) inhibiting the use of glucose in the peripheral tissues and (2) inducing hepatic synthesis of enzymes involved in gluconeogenesis. In addition, these drugs predispose the patient to developing posterior subcapsular cataracts; the mechanism for this action, however, is somewhat unclear.

56. (**A**) A renal contusion is the most probable result of blunt injuries to the kidney. Also, the fact that the renal collecting system has not been damaged, as is evidenced by the urine output and specific gravity, rules out all of the other possibilities.

67. The most appropriate nursing interventions to use in caring for a patient experiencing hyponatremia due to sodium depletion would be to

    A. Monitor intake and output and give diuretics as prescribed.
    B. Monitor neurologic status and give .25 NS I.V. as prescribed.
    C. Monitor respiratory status and give .45 NS I.V. as prescribed.
    D. Monitor urine sodium levels and give a high-sodium diet.

68. Which of the following is a likely complication of chronic hypercalcemia?

    A. Laryngeal stridor.
    B. Renal calculi.
    C. Psychoses.
    D. Seizures.

69. A patient with a serum calcium of 12.0 mg/dl is likely to be treated using which of the following?

    A. Vitamin D and phosphate.
    B. Corticosteroids and loop diuretics.
    C. Amphojel and mithramycin.
    D. Rocaltrol and sodium bicarbonate.

70. A patient with a serum calcium level of 7.0 mg/dl is likely to exhibit which of the following sets of signs and symptoms?

    A. Paresthesias and muscle cramps.
    B. Constipation and abdominal cramps.
    C. Tetany and polyuria.
    D. Deep bone pain and depression.

71. Which of the following nursing interventions are appropriate in the care of a patient who is experiencing hypocalcemia?

    A. Monitor Trousseau's sign and give eggs.
    B. Monitor output and give cheese.
    C. Monitor the central nervous system status and give sodium bicarbonate as prescribed.
    D. Check Chvostek's sign and give vitamin D as prescribed.

57. (C) If renal function is normal, the results of the traumatic injury would be manifested in the serum by the accumulation of the waste products of catabolism, which would reflect the destruction of normal tissues. In addition, a decrease in fluid volume would further increase the BUN level.

58. (B) When urine leaks or is forced into the abdominal cavity, a number of potential problems may occur, including infection, renal failure, and further abdominal trauma. Thus, the problem must be surgically corrected as soon as possible.

59. (C) Bedrest will assist in decreasing the hematuria and traumatic effects on the kidney. Analgesics will decrease the pain associated with stretching of the renal capsule by the contusion. The patient's fluid intake should be normal, and surgical intervention is usually not indicated for renal contusions.

60. (D) Hyperkalemia increases gastric motility and produces diarrhea. It also produces flaccid paralysis by partially depolarizing the muscle-cell membrane and then blocking further depolarization.

61. (C) Kayexalate is a cation exchange resin that exchanges sodium ions for potassium ions in the gastrointestinal tract. The potassium ions are then excreted through the feces, and total body potassium levels decrease. All of the other measures alter the membrane effects of hyperkalemia or affect the transcellular movement of potassium but do not decrease the total body potassium levels.

62. (A) Hypokalemia decreases gastric motility to such an extent that a paralytic ileus occurs. The major complication following a paralytic ileus is that of perforation. All of the other complications are unrelated to a hypokalemic state.

72. The following set of serum laboratory values were obtained from a patient on your unit:

Na 140 mEq/L   Ca 6.0 mg/dl
K 5.0 mEq/L   PO$_4$ 8.0 mg/dl
Cl 101 mEq/L   Mg 1.0 mEq/L

Which electrolyte imbalances would you expect the patient to exhibit?

A. Hyperkalemia, hyperchloremia, and hyperphosphatemia.
B. Hypocalcemia, hyperkalemia, and hypermagnesemia.
C. Hypocalcemia, hyperphosphatemia, and hypomagnesemia.
D. Hyperchloremia, hypernatremia, and hypermagnesemia.

73. Which of the following nursing interventions would be appropriate in caring for a patient with a serum phosphate of 1.6 mg/dl?

A. Assist with ADL's and give milk.
B. Monitor Trousseau's sign and give eggs.
C. Provide a safe environment and give vitamin D as prescribed.
D. Assess muscle strength and give hard American cheese.

Answers to Questions from page 102

63. (C) Intake and output should be monitored in order to accurately assess the effects of the polyuria that is induced by the hypokalemia. Raisins are given because they are an excellent source of potassium. One cup of raisins contains about 30 mEq of potassium.

64. (D) Normal serum values for these substances are:

Na 136–145 mEq/L   Ca 8.5–10.5 mg/dl
K 3.5–5.5 mEq/L   PO$_4$ 3.0–4.5 mg/dl
Cl 96–106 mEq/L   Mg 1.5–2.5 mEq/L

65. (A) Patients experiencing hypernatremia due to excessive water loss have very dry mucous membranes and are very thirsty. Oral hygiene helps to alleviate those symptoms. The excessive water loss needs to be replaced slowly using a .45 NS solution to avoid creating rebound hyponatremia.

66. (B) For each 100 mg of increase in glucose there is a 2 mEq/L decrease in serum sodium because of the shift of water from the intracellular to the extracellular space secondary to the hyperglycemia. Thus, states of hyperglycemia can easily create hyponatremia. The other etiologies will produce hypernatremia, *not* hyponatremia.

74. A patient with a serum magnesium of 12.0 mEq/L would exhibit which of the following signs and symptoms?

   A. Hypoventilation and coma.
   B. Hyperreflexia and hypotension.
   C. Sinus tachycardia and muscle weakness.
   D. Vomiting and hypertension.

75. Which of the following conditions is a major cause of hypomagnesemia in critically ill patients?

   A. Alkalosis.
   B. Prolonged hyperalimentation therapy.
   C. Hypervolemia.
   D. Decreased aldosterone secretion.

Answers to Questions from page 103

67. (**D**) The urine sodium is usually less than 10 mEq/L in hyponatremic states due to sodium deficit. Continuous monitoring will assist in assessing the adequacy of replacement therapy. Replacement therapy would usually consist of a high-sodium diet and/or at least .9 NS I.V.

68. (**B**) Renal calculi are a common complication of chronic hypercalcemia because of the increased urinary excretion of calcium that occurs as a compensatory mechanism.

69. (**B**) Corticosteroids decrease the gastrointestinal reabsorption of calcium, and loop diuretics increase the urinary calcium excretion rate. Phosphate, mithramycin, and sodium bicarbonate will also assist in decreasing serum calcium levels. However, the other measures will only increase the serum calcium levels.

70. (**A**) The effects of low calcium on the neuromuscular system are such that they increase the neuron permeability and cause irritability. Abdominal cramps, tetany, and depression also signify hypocalcemia. The other signs and symptoms indicate hypercalcemia.

71. (**D**) Checking Chvostek's sign is one way of assessing for decreased serum levels of calcium. Giving vitamin D will increase the gastrointestinal reabsorption of calcium. Monitoring Trousseau's sign, giving cheese, and monitoring the central nervous system status are also acceptable interventions. However, giving eggs or sodium bicarbonate would only further decrease the calcium level. Also, there is no valid reason to monitor the urinary output in hypocalcemic states.

72. (**C**) Normal serum values for these substances are:

Na 136–145 mEq/L   Ca 8.5–10.5 mg/dl
K 3.5–5.5 mEq/L PO_4 3.0–4.5 mg/dl
Cl 96–106 mEq/L   Mg 1.5–2.5 mEq/L

73. (**D**) Hypophosphatemia decreases the energy available to cells and results in muscle weakness. Cheese is higher in phosphate than it is in calcium and acts as an excellent source for replacement. Eggs are also high in phosphate; milk, however, is higher in calcium than in phosphate, so it is not a good replacement substance. Assisting with ADLs and providing a safe environment are also valid nursing interventions for a hypophosphatemic patient. The other interventions, however, relate to hypocalcemic states.

74. (**A**) Magnesium levels greater than 10.0 mEq/L have a severe depressive effect on all muscles, resulting in paralysis, hypoventilation, and coma. Hypotension, vomiting, and muscle weakness also accompany hypermagnesemia; however, they appear at much lower levels.

75. (**B**) Most hyperalimentation solutions are relatively deficient in magnesium. Thus, if magnesium is not replaced periodically, the patient becomes hypomagnesemic.

Bibliography

American Association of Critical-Care Nurses: Core Curriculum for Critical Care Nursing, 3rd ed. W. B. Saunders Co., Philadelphia, 1985.
An overview of essential information concerning critical care nursing practice. Presented in a systems framework utilizing an outline format.

Brundage, D. J.: Nursing Management of Renal Problems, 2nd ed. C. V. Mosby Co., St. Louis, 1980.
A concise overview of renal function, dysfunction, and therapeutic interventions. The book is divided into two major sections, the conservation of renal function and the restoration of renal function. Presents a nice review of the components involved in the continuum of renal function to renal failure.

Drukker, W., Parsons, F. M., and Maher, J. F.: Replacement of Renal Function by Dialysis, 2nd ed. Martinus Nijhoff Publishers, Boston, 1983.
An excellent in-depth approach to dialysis therapy. Covers all aspects involved, including the principles, structure, kinetics, complications, access sites, and much more. One of the most comprehensive texts on this topic. Probably not for the novice clinician.

Early, L. E., and Gottschalk, C. W.: Strauss and Welt's Diseases of the Kidney, 3rd ed. Little, Brown and Co., Boston, 1979.
A comprehensive, two-volume set of works devoted to the normal function of the kidney, renal failure and its consequences and management, various categories of renal pathology, the effects of other systemic diseases on the kidney, and disorders of water and electrolyte metabolism. Most of the discussions are in-depth approaches.

Friedman, E. A. (ed.): Strategy in Renal Failure. John Wiley & Sons, Inc., New York, 1978.
A discussion of renal failure—its manifestations and management strategies. Some excellent content related to the psychosocial, financial, and governmental aspects of renal failure. A classic work in the area of managing renal failure patients.

Hamburger, J., Crosnier, J., and Grunfeld, J. P. (eds.): Nephrology. John Wiley & Sons, Inc., New York, 1979.
A comprehensive text covering all aspects of nephrology. Best used for isolated topics rather than read from cover to cover. Some good in-depth physiologic discussions and explanations.

Klahr, S.: Differential Diagnosis: Renal and Electrolyte Disorders. Arco Publishing Co., New York, 1978.
A nice signs and symptoms approach to fluid, electrolyte, and acid-base disorders. Excellent physiologic interpretations and good illustrating case studies. Definitely a clinician's approach to patient care from the medical perspective.

Lancaster, L. E. (ed.): The Patient with End Stage Renal Disease, 2nd ed. John Wiley & Sons, Inc., New York, 1984.
A comprehensive approach to caring for the individual with end stage renal disease. Covers all facets of management. Probably the best text from a nursing perspective on this topic. Excellent for students and clinicians.

Leaf, A., and Cotran, R.: Renal Pathophysiology. Oxford University Press, New York, 1976.
A concise overview of renal physiology and pathophysiology. Excellent physiologic discussions using case studies to illustrate major points.

Kinney, M. R., Dear, C. B., Packa, D. R., and Voorman, D. M. N. (eds.): AACN's Clinical Reference for Critical-Care Nursing. McGraw-Hill Book Co., New York, 1981.
A comprehensive approach to critical care nursing. Includes the conceptual foundations, the physiologic bases, physical assessment, the psychosocial bases, dynamic system interrelationships, patient care management, procedures and principles, the environment, ethical issues, and patient teaching and rehabilitation. Perhaps a classic in critical care nursing.

Schrier, R. W. (ed.): Renal and Electrolyte Disorders, 2nd. ed. Little, Brown and Co., Boston, 1980.
An excellent in-depth approach to fluid and electrolyte disorders. The physiologic discussions are concrete and very useful for clinicians. Certainly one of the best books on this topic.

Stein, J. H. (ed.): Nephrology. Grune & Stratton, New York, 1980.
A comprehensive overview of nephrology including anatomy, histology, normal function, hormonal actions, diagnostic methods, clinical syndromes and symptoms, imbalances, specific diseases, and treatment. A good book for clinicians, but not for novices.

Valtin, H.: Renal dysfunction: Mechanisms Involved in Fluid and Solute Imbalance. Little, Brown and Co., Boston, 1979.
An excellent book for clinicians. Good physiologic discussions with ample illustrations. Includes case studies and problems to facilitate learning. Great for the advanced learner.

Valtin, H.: Renal Function: Mechanisms Preserving Fluid and Solute Balance in Health. Little, Brown and Co., Boston, 1973.
An excellent physiologic text. Perhaps prerequisite to his previously listed text. Includes chapters on the components of renal function, body fluid compartments, glomerular filtration, tubular reabsorption and secretion, hemodynamics and oxygen consumption, sodium transport, concentration and dilution, hydrogen balance, and renal handling of hydrogen and potassium. Also has study problems to enhance learning.

Vander, A. J.: Renal Physiology. McGraw-Hill Book Co., New York, 1975.
A succinct but thorough presentation of renal physiology. Contains learning objectives and lots of illustrations. Great for the student or new clinician.

5 □ THE ENDOCRINE SYSTEM

TERESA THOMA KEVIL
SUSAN ARMSTRONG SCREWS

1. The anterior pituitary functions in response to releasing and inhibiting hormones/factors secreted by the

   A. Hypothalamus.
   B. Posterior pituitary.
   C. Adrenal medulla.
   D. Adrenal cortex.

2. A rise in the circulating level of most hormones inhibits their further production. This mechanism of regulating hormonal secretion rate is known as

   A. Autonomy.
   B. Positive feedback.
   C. Negative feedback.
   D. Diurnal variation.

3. Posterior pituitary secretions are controlled by the hypothalamus via what type of connection?

   A. Vascular.
   B. Neural.
   C. Muscular.
   D. Lymphatic.

4. Secretion of growth hormone is inhibited by

   A. Hypoglycemia.
   B. L-Dopa.
   C. Glucagon.
   D. Somatostatin.

5. Tropic hormones are those that stimulate glandular secretion. Which of the following is *not* a tropic hormone?

   A. ACTH.
   B. TSH.
   C. FSH.
   D. GH.

6. Corticotropin (ACTH) is secreted by the

   A. Anterior pituitary.
   B. Posterior pituitary.
   C. Hypothalamus.
   D. Adrenal cortex.

7. A rise in ACTH in response to stress is stimulated by a

   A. Negative feedback mechanism.
   B. Circadian variation.
   C. Hypothalamic releasing factor.
   D. Posterior pituitary hormone.

8. The major function of ACTH is to stimulate release of

   A. Vasopressin.
   B. Cortisol.
   C. Growth inhibiting hormone.
   D. Thyroid stimulating hormone.

9. Release of thyrotropin (TSH) is stimulated by

   A. Hypothalamic releasing factor.
   B. Somatostatin.
   C. Anxiety.
   D. Increased levels of thyroid hormone.

10. Vasopressin is produced by the

    A. Hypothalamus.
    B. Anterior pituitary.
    C. Posterior pituitary.
    D. Adrenal cortex.

11. The primary action of antidiuretic hormone is to

    A. Promote sodium and water reabsorption in the renal tubules.
    B. Stimulate the release of cortisol from the adrenal cortex.
    C. Stimulate adrenal cortical cells to produce aldosterone.
    D. Promote water reabsorption in the distal tubules and collecting ducts.

12. Which of the following diseases is characterized by deficient ADH secretion?

    A. Syndrome of inappropriate ADH.
    B. Diabetes insipidus.
    C. Cushing's syndrome.
    D. Addison's disease.

13. The hormone secreted in response to genital tract distention and uterine contractions is

    A. Luteinizing hormone.
    B. Follicle stimulating hormone.
    C. Oxytocin.
    D. Prolactin.

14. Which of the following statements regarding triiodothyronine (T_3) *is true*?

    A. It accounts for about 90% of the thyroid hormone released.
    B. It is more potent and has a shorter duration than T_4.
    C. It is converted to T_4 in the periphery.
    D. It is synthesized by parafollicular cells in the thyroid.

15. One of the physiologic effects of T_3 and T_4 is to

    A. Decrease metabolism in all body cells.
    B. Increase cellular oxygen consumption.
    C. Decrease metabolism of protein.
    D. Antagonize growth hormones.

16. The primary task of parathormone is to increase serum calcium ion levels. Another hormone that plays a lesser role in reducing serum calcium ion levels is

    A. 1,25-Dihydroxycholecalciferol.
    B. Cortisol.
    C. Thyrocalcitonin.
    D. Dehydroepiandrosterone.

17. Somatostatin is secreted by delta cells in the

    A. Liver.
    B. Adrenals.
    C. Kidneys.
    D. Pancreas.

18. Which of the following is *not* a physiological effect of insulin?

    A. It increases gluconeogenesis in the liver.
    B. It increases the transport of glucose across some cell membranes.
    C. It increases triglyceride and protein synthesis.
    D. It has a synergistic effect on growth hormones.

Answers to Questions from page 109

1. **(A)** Function of the anterior pituitary is regulated by hypothalamic hormones. These chemical factors are carried from the hypothalamus to the pituitary via vascular connections (portal hypophyseal vessels).

2. **(C)** The secretion rate of some hormones is aligned with body need via a negative feedback mechanism. One example is the control of cortisol secretion. Release of cortisol is regulated by ACTH. When cortisol levels fall, ACTH levels rise, thus increasing the rate of cortisol secretion. Increased cortisol levels then feed back to inhibit ACTH secretion.

3. **(B)** The hypothalamus controls secretions of the posterior pituitary by direct neural connection. Posterior pituitary hormones are synthesized in nerve cell bodies in the hypothalamus, and then travel along the nerve (supraopticohypophyseal) axons to the posterior pituitary, where they are stored in the nerve endings until released into circulation.

4. **(D)** Somatostatin, a hypothalamic inhibiting factor, inhibits the release of somatotropin (growth hormone). Secretion is also inhibited by hyperglycemia. All other factors listed above stimulate release of growth hormone.

5. **(D)** Growth hormone stimulates cell growth throughout the body. Since it does not stimulate the release of a substance from any gland, GH is not a tropic hormone. Tropic hormones include TSH, ACTH, FSH, and LH.

6. **(A)** ACTH is an anterior pituitary hormone. Others include somatotropin, prolactin, TSH, FSH, and LH.

19. Glucagon release by the pancreas is inhibited by insulin, somatostatin, and

    A. Hypoglycemia.
    B. Hypokalemia.
    C. Hyperglycemia.
    D. Hypercalcemia.

20. Two weeks after bilateral adrenalectomy, a patient has developed an upper respiratory infection. Which of the following is most critical to her survival?

    A. Administering ACTH.
    B. Initiating gentamycin therapy.
    C. Placing her in protective isolation and restricting visitors to her immediate family.
    D. Increasing her exogenous intake of synthetic glucocorticoids.

21. Which of the following physiologic effects can be due to the administration of large amounts of glucocorticoids?

    A. Stabilization of lysosomal membranes.
    B. Increased protein anabolism.
    C. Increased glucose utilization in the periphery.
    D. Increased protein stores in all body cells, especially the liver.

22. Which of the following hormones is most essential for controlling serum potassium ion concentration?

    A. Cortisol.
    B. Aldosterone.
    C. Vasopressin.
    D. Parathormone.

23. The catecholamines, epinephrine and norepinephrine, are secreted by the

    A. Adrenal cortex.
    B. Posterior pituitary.
    C. Hypothalamus.
    D. Adrenal medulla.

24. The effects of catecholamines on $beta_2$ receptors include

    A. Generalized vasoconstriction.
    B. Negative chronotropic effect on the heart.
    C. Bronchoconstriction.
    D. Vasodilation in skeletal and cardiac muscle.

Answers to Questions from page 110

7. (**C**) Corticotropin releasing factor (CRF) from the hypothalamus stimulates the release of ACTH in response to stress. This occurs independent of, and may supercede secretion regulation by, diurnal variation and feedback.

8. (**B**) ACTH controls the secretion of cortisol from the adrenal cortex. Cortisol then feeds back to control ACTH secretion.

9. (**A**) Thyrotropin is released in response to thyrotropin releasing hormone (TRH) from the hypothalamus. Decreased circulating levels of thyroid hormone stimulate release via the feedback mechanism. TSH secretion is inhibited by increased levels of thyroid hormone, somatostatin, and possibly some emotions.

10. (**A**) Vasopressin, or antidiuretic hormone (ADH), is synthesized within cell bodies of the hypothalamus. The hormone is then transported down axons to the posterior pituitary. The hormone is secreted in response to neural impulses from the hypothalamus.

11. (**D**) ADH promotes water reabsorption in the distal tubules and collecting ducts. Aldosterone promotes sodium and water reabsorption in the renal tubules. Adrenocorticotropic hormone stimulates the release of cortisol from the adrenal cortex. Angiotensin II stimulates adrenal cortical cells to produce aldosterone.

12. (**B**) ADH secretion is deficient in diabetes insipidus because of inflammatory cerebral edema or direct damage to the hypothalamus. The syndrome of inappropriate ADH secretion is associated with excessive ADH secretion. Cushing's syndrome results from increased production of cortisol by the adrenal gland. Addison's disease is primary adrenocortical deficiency.

25. When eliciting a health history from a patient with a possible endocrine disorder, the nurse should

    A. Keep the interview brief.
    B. Make sure the history is detailed.
    C. Avoid taking notes.
    D. Have the patient lie down.

26. *Hirsutism* is defined as the presence of

    A. A male pattern of hair distribution.
    B. An abnormal muscle enlargement.
    C. A male body habitus.
    D. Multiple masculinizing features.

27. A normal finding on assessment of the thyroid gland is

    A. Tenderness.
    B. Nodular consistency.
    C. Marked asymmetry.
    D. Movements on swallowing.

28. Which of the following may be an unrealistic goal in planning nursing care for a patient with endocrine dysfunction?

    A. The patient will be able to regain/maintain normal metabolism.
    B. The patient and family will be able to verbalize knowledge of self-care practices necessary to prevent endocrine crises from recurring.
    C. The patient will be independent of pharmacologic agents by discharge.
    D. The patient will be able to engage in activities of daily living.

29. When teaching self-care information to the patient and/or family, which of the following should the nurse do first?

    A. Establish outcome criteria.
    B. Assess the patient's learning needs and readiness.
    C. Record patient response to teaching.
    D. Develop a topical outline of what will be presented.

30. The nurse should recognize that diagnostic findings associated with diabetes insipidus include

    A. Increased urine osmolality.
    B. Elevated serum glucose.
    C. Decreased urine specific gravity.
    D. Presence of urine ketones.

Answers to Questions from page 111

13. (**C**) Oxytocin is secreted from the posterior pituitary in response to genital tract distention, to uterine contractions, and also to suckling. The effects of oxytocin are to eject milk from the secretory ducts and to contract uterine smooth muscle. Luteinizing hormone (LH) and follicle stimulating hormone (FSH) are secreted by the anterior pituitary in response to specific hypothalamic releasing factors. Secretion of prolactin by the anterior pituitary is regulated by prolactin inhibitory factor (PIF) from the hypothalamus.

14. (**B**) Triiodothyronine (T_3) is more potent and has a shorter duration than thyroxine (T_4). T_3 accounts for about 10%, and T_4 for about 90%, of the thyroid hormone released from the thyroid gland. T_4 is converted to T_3 in the periphery. Both T_4 and T_3 are synthesized in the thyroid follicles.

15. (**B**) Physiologically, T_3 and T_4 increase cellular oxygen consumption. They also increase metabolism in almost all body cells, stimulate metabolism of carbohydrates, fats, and protein, and potentiate growth hormones.

16. (**C**) Thyrocalcitonin, or calcitonin, is synthesized by parafollicular cells in the thyroid gland. It plays a small role in reducing serum calcium ion levels by inhibiting bone resorption and interfering with the formation of active vitamin D (1,25-dihydroxycholecalciferol). Cortisol is a glucocorticoid released by the adrenal cortex. Dehydroepiandrosterone is an adrenal androgen.

17. (**D**) Somatostatin is secreted by delta cells in the pancreas. It can also be found in other areas, such as the hypothalamus and gastrointestinal tract. Insulin is produced by pancreatic beta cells, and glucagon is produced by pancreatic alpha cells.

18. (**A**) Insulin inhibits gluconeogenesis in the liver, but it increases liver synthesis of glycogen.

31. Appropriate nursing actions related to the administration of vasopressin tannate in oil include all *except*

    A. Warm solution.
    B. Shake vigorously.
    C. Administer intramuscularly.
    D. Administer before previous dose has worn off.

32. Which of the following should the nurse recognize as a sign of water intoxication?

    A. Hiccoughs.
    B. Headache.
    C. Increased body temperature.
    D. Flank pain.

33. Routine nursing measures appropriate for the diabetes insipidus patient include all *except*

    A. Accurate intake and output.
    B. Restricted oral fluids.
    C. Daily weights.
    D. Encouraged rest periods.

34. The purpose of administering chlorpropamide (Diabinese) to patients with diabetes insipidus is to

    A. Lower serum glucose.
    B. Potentiate vasopressin.
    C. Inhibit potassium loss.
    D. Induce diuresis.

35. The syndrome of inappropriate ADH secretion (SIADH) is characterized by plasma

    A. Hypertonicity and hyponatremia.
    B. Hypertonicity and hypernatremia.
    C. Hypotonicity and hyponatremia.
    D. Hypotonicity and hypernatremia.

36. All of the following are etiologically associated with SIADH *except*

    A. Pharmacologic agents.
    B. Central nervous system disorders.
    C. Intrathoracic disorders.
    D. Renal disorders.

Answers to Questions from page 112

19. (**C**) An increase in blood glucose will inhibit the release of glucagon from alpha cells in the pancreas.

20. (**D**) In normal adrenal function, the body responds to stress by increasing secretion of ACTH from the anterior pituitary, leading to increased secretion of glucocorticoids. If the patient is unable to elevate cortisol levels endogenously in response to stress such as infection, then it is essential that exogenous ingestion be appropriately altered. Because steroids mask signs of infection, it is important to monitor closely for infection and, when it is present, to culture organisms to identify appropriate antimicrobial therapy.

21. (**A**) Large amounts of glucocorticoids have been found to stabilize lysosomal membranes. This stabilization contributes to an anti-inflammatory effect. Glucocorticoids increase protein catabolism or breakdown, decrease glucose utilization in the periphery, and can cause an insulin-resistant diabetes. They also decrease protein stores in all body cells for diversion to the liver, where stores are increased.

22. (**B**) Aldosterone is integral in the regulation of potassium ion concentration. It increases the rate of tubular reabsorption of sodium. The electronegativity in the tubules then attracts potassium. The net effect of aldosterone is the retention of sodium and the excretion of potassium. The level of potassium ion concentration regulates secretion of aldosterone, as does the renin-angiotensin system.

23. (**D**) The catecholamines are secreted by the adrenal medulla. They are regulated by direct nervous system control and are the first line of defense against stress.

24. (**D**) The effects of catecholamines on beta$_2$ receptors include vasodilation in skeletal and cardiac muscle, bronchodilation, and glycogenolysis. Catecholamine effects on alpha receptors include generalized vasoconstriction, intestinal and bladder sphincter contraction, and decreased insulin secretion. Their effects on beta$_1$ receptors include positive chronotropic and inotropic effects on the heart.

37. The clinical presentation of SIADH may include

    A. Confusion.
    B. Dependent edema.
    C. Weight loss.
    D. Polyphagia.

38. The nurse should expect a patient with SIADH to exhibit decreased

    A. Plasma osmolality.
    B. Urine specific gravity.
    C. Urine osmolality.
    D. Ability to retain water.

39. Which of the following nursing interventions would most likely be instituted in the acute phase for the patient with SIADH?

    A. Force fluids and give I.V. furosemide to stimulate diuresis.
    B. Limit fluid intake to 1000 ml NS over 24 hours.
    C. Restrict fluid intake to urine output plus insensible losses.
    D. Restrict total fluid intake to 2 L per 24 hours.

40. Thyrotoxic crisis is a life-threatening emergency characterized by a fulminating increase in the signs and symptoms of

    A. Hypothyroidism.
    B. Hyperthyroidism.
    C. Myxedema.
    D. Euthyroidism.

41. Which of the following symptoms should the nurse recognize as characteristic of thyrotoxic crisis?

    A. Bradycardia.
    B. Extreme flaccidity.
    C. Bradypnea.
    D. Hyperthermia.

42. Physical examination findings consistent with thyrotoxic crisis include

    A. A bruit over the thyroid gland.
    B. Narrowed pulse pressure.
    C. Nonpalpable thyroid gland.
    D. Pulmonary consolidation.

Answers to Questions from page 113

25. (**B**) Endocrinologic disorders may result in variations in virtually all body systems. The health history must be thorough, including detailed past, present, and family history. Each positive finding should be explored in terms of onset, intensity, duration, associated manifestations, and precipitating and alleviating factors. Note-taking assures accurate recording of data.

26. (**A**) Abnormal hair distribution in the male pattern is hirsutism. Often associated with increased androgen levels, hirsutism may be accompanied by other masculinizing features.

27. (**B**) The thyroid is a butterfly-shaped gland positioned over the trachea below the cricoid cartilage. The lobes, if palpable, are normally smooth and tender. The right and left lobes are approximately equal in size, although slight asymmetry is often found.

28. (**C**) It may be unrealistic to expect a patient with endocrine dysfunction to be independent of drugs by discharge. Many patients are diagnosed as having chronic conditions that will require medication for the rest of their lives. It is the responsibility of the nurse to insure that the patient and/or family fully understands the importance of compliance and the consequences of noncompliance.

29. (**B**) The first step to take when teaching a patient is to assess the patient's learning needs and his learning readiness. Assessment is the first step in the nursing process. The second step in the process, planning, would include such things as establishing outcome criteria and developing a topical outline. A part of the third step, implementation, would involve providing instruction and noting the patient's response to teaching. The last step in the nursing process is evaluation, in which the nurse evaluates the effectiveness of teaching.

30. (**C**) Diabetes insipidus is a disorder in which the kidneys are unable to concentrate urine. The urine is greatly increased in volume, with lower osmolality and specific gravity. Diabetes insipidus is not a disorder of glucose metabolism.

43. Diagnostic findings in hyperthyroid crisis may include

    A. Decreased total and free T_3 and T_4.
    B. Decreased T_3 resin uptake.
    C. Severe hypoglycemia.
    D. Atrial fibrillation.

44. Which of the following pharmacologic agents is *not* recommended for treating hyperthyroid crisis?

    A. Propylthiouracil.
    B. Propranolol.
    C. Glucocorticoids.
    D. Aspirin.

45. A 64-year-old female is brought to the emergency room in a somnolent state. Pertinent data include: T 96°F; P 50; R 8 per minute; BP 84/56; Pa_{O_2} 50; Pa_{CO_2} 55. Her symptomatology is consistent with

    A. Impending hyperthyroid crisis.
    B. Impending myxedema coma.
    C. Addison's disease.
    D. Crohn's disease.

46. Myxedema coma is a life-threatening emergency characterized by exaggerated signs and symptoms of severe

    A. Adrenal insufficiency.
    B. Hyperthyroidism.
    C. Hypothyroidism.
    D. Renal disease.

47. Which of the following symptoms would a patient with chronic hypothyroidism most likely exhibit?

    A. Rapid relaxation phase of deep tendon reflexes.
    B. Cold intolerance.
    C. Polyphagia.
    D. Diarrhea.

Answers to Questions from page 114

31. (**D**) Vasopressin tannate in oil, as many oil preparations, should be warmed prior to administration to enhance patient comfort and facilitate administration. Because the active hormone settles in oil, vigorous shaking is necessary before administration. This drug is readministered after polyuria and polydipsia return, allowing excretion of excess free water. Effects last up to 48 hours.

32. (**B**) Signs of water intoxication include nausea, drowsiness, and headache. Water intoxication should be observed for when exogenous vasopressin is being administered to a patient with chronic polydipsia.

33. (**B**) Adequate fluids should be provided to prevent dehydration. Oral fluids may be restricted for specified periods of time only as part of a diagnostic evaluation.

34. (**B**) Diabinese is given to potentiate vasopressin. Patients should be instructed concerning the possibility of hypoglycemic reaction.

35. (**C**) In SIADH, antidiuretic hormone continues to be secreted in spite of low plasma osmolality and increased volume. Water intoxication results in dilutional hyponatremia. There is also commonly an inability to dilute the urine, leading to plasma hypotonicity and urinary hypertonicity. Urine may sometimes be hypotonic, but it is not as dilute as would be expected in these circumstances.

36. (**D**) Causes of SIADH include malignancies, nonmalignant pulmonary disorders (including the use of positive-pressure ventilation), central nervous system disorders, and pharmacologic agents. Although renal disorders may manifest similar symptomatology, they are not accompanied by elevated plasma ADH levels.

48. Most of the serious complications that can occur secondary to myxedema coma involve the respiratory system and the

   A. Cardiovascular system.
   B. Renal system.
   C. Neuromuscular system.
   D. Gastrointestinal system.

49. Of the following admission orders for a patient in myxedema coma, which should the nurse question before giving?

   A. Levothyroxine 0.3 mg I.V. push now.
   B. Hydrocortisone 50 mg I.V.P.B. q 6 h.
   C. Infuse 1000 ml $D_5\frac{1}{2}NS$ at 12 h rate.
   D. Percodan one tab q 6 h PRN pain.

50. In a patient with myxedema coma, which of the following findings should the nurse interpret as a positive response to medical treatment?

   A. An increase in body temperature.
   B. A rapid rise in Pa_{CO_2}.
   C. A decrease in arterial pH.
   D. An increase in body weight.

51. Which of the following nursing interventions is of primary importance to the stable patient with chronic thyroid dysfunction?

   A. Perform all activities of daily living for the patient.
   B. Restrict visitors.
   C. Initiate self-care education for the patient and family.
   D. Provide constant environmental stimulation.

Answers to Questions from page 115

37. (A) Patients with SIADH may present with fatigue, headache, weakness, and restlessness. They may exhibit personality changes, mental confusion, lethargy, irritability, and sluggish deep tendon reflexes, as well as some weight gain due to water intoxication with or without evidence of edema. Nausea, vomiting, diarrhea, and anorexia may also be seen. If the hyponatremia becomes severe enough, convulsions and/or coma may develop.

38. (A) Plasma osmolality is decreased in SIADH because of excessive water retention. Concomitantly, there are frequently increases in urine osmolality and urinary specific gravity. In some instances, urine may be hypotonic or not as dilute as it should be.

39. (C) Oral and parenteral fluids are generally restricted to replacement of urine output plus insensible losses (frequently in the range of 500 to 1000 ml daily). With life-threatening hyponatremia, hypertonic saline is administered to elevate the serum sodium to levels at which symptoms improve. I.V. furosemide may be given concomitantly to reduce the risk of developing congestive heart failure secondary to fluid overload. Its administration necessitates careful monitoring and replacement of electrolytes, such as potassium.

40. (B) Thyrotoxic crisis presents as a fulminating increase in the signs and symptoms of thyrotoxicosis, or hyperthyroidism. Myxedema is an advanced form of hypothyroidism. *Euthyroidism* refers to a normal thyroid state.

41. (D) Fever to 106°F or more, tachycardia, tachypnea, nausea, vomiting, diarrhea, tremors, extreme irritability, psychosis, and coma are all characteristic symptoms of thyrotoxic crisis.

42. (A) In thyrotoxic crisis, physical examination may reveal a bruit and thrill over the thyroid gland. The thyroid gland is palpable and enlarged. Patients demonstrate a widened pulse pressure.

52. Dysfunction of the parathyroid glands and parathormone production results in alterations in calcium and

    A. Potassium.
    B. Phosphate.
    C. Sodium.
    D. Chloride.

53. In primary adrenal insufficiency, the nurse should anticipate deficiency of

    A. Glucocorticoids only.
    B. Mineralocorticoids only.
    C. Glucocorticoids and mineralocorticoids.
    D. Adrenocorticotropic hormone.

54. One of the physical findings that helps distinguish primary from secondary adrenal insufficiency is

    A. Hyperpigmentation of the skin.
    B. Vomiting.
    C. Muscle weakness.
    D. Abdominal pain.

55. Which of the following fluid and electrolyte disorders would most likely occur in adrenal crisis?

    A. Hypernatremia.
    B. Hyperkalemia.
    C. Hypervolemia.
    D. Hyperchloremia.

43. (**D**) ECG findings in hyperthyroid crisis may include sinus tachycardia, atrial fibrillation, premature ventricular contractions, and premature atrial contractions. Elevations in total and free T_3 and T_4 levels as well as T_3 resin uptake are also seen. Hyperglycemia may occur because of insulin resistance, impaired insulin secretion, or increased glycogenolysis. Owing to the hypermetabolic state of hyperthyroid crisis, some patients may get mildly hypoglycemic from metabolism of gluocse.

44. (**D**) Aspirin is not recommended for reducing fever because it displaces T_3 from its carrier protein, causing an increase in free T_3 levels. Propylthiouracil inhibits hormone synthesis and prevents the conversion of T_4 to T_3 in the periphery. Propranolol, a beta-adrenergic blocker, will decrease peripheral effects and may block conversion of T_4 to T_3. Glucocorticoids, which may also block the conversion of T_4 to T_3, are given to offset adrenal insufficiency and decreased adrenal reserve in these patients.

45. (**B**) A patient in myxedema coma may present with profound hypothermia, hypoventilation with resulting hypoxemia and hypercapnia, hypotension, bradycardia, seizures, and coma. Addison's disease results from a deficiency in the secretion of adrenocortical hormones. Crohn's disease is a chronic inflammatory condition of the bowel.

46. (**C**) Myxedema coma results from extreme hypothyroidism, in which there is an accumulation of a mucopolysaccharide substance. Clinical manifestations of myxedema may demonstrate involvement of the skin, vocal cords, middle ear, or vital organs.

47. (**B**) Patients with chronic hypothyroidism may exhibit cold intolerance, delayed return of deep tendon reflexes, weight gain despite anorexia, constipation, hoarseness, mood changes, bradycardia, subcutaneous swelling, and menstrual irregularities.

56. In caring for a patient in adrenal crisis, which nursing intervention would be most appropriate?

   A. Withhold glucocorticoid preparations until the crisis has passed.
   B. Perform activities of daily living for the patient.
   C. Encourage ingestion of high-potassium, low-sodium foods and fluids.
   D. Allow more frequent visits by members of the patient's family.

57. Diabetic ketoacidosis (DKA) occurs as a result of

   A. Insulin overdose.
   B. Insulin deficiency.
   C. Increased tissue glucose.
   D. Insulin releasing factor deficiency.

58. *Gluconeogenesis* is the formation of glucose from

   A. Carbohydrate.
   B. Noncarbohydrate sources.
   C. Glycogen.
   D. Fat.

59. In DKA, the energy for gluconeogenesis is supplied primarily by

   A. Breakdown of amino acids.
   B. Release of hepatic enzymes.
   C. Circulating glucose.
   D. Oxidation of fatty acids.

60. Insulin therapy for diabetic ketoacidosis results in which of the following changes?

   A. Increased cellular potassium.
   B. Decreased cellular potassium.
   C. Increased serum glucose.
   D. Increased serum potassium.

61. Factors that may precipitate diabetic ketoacidosis include

   A. Weight reduction.
   B. Exercise.
   C. Stress.
   D. Low-carbohydrate diet.

Answers to Questions from page 117

48. (**A**) Aside from possible respiratory complications of respiratory failure and pleural effusion, serious cardiovascular complications may occur, such as pericardial effusion, accelerated atherosclerosis, circulatory overload, and cardiovascular collapse. Gastrointestinal complications include adynamic ileus. The mortality rate from these complications is near 50%.

49. (**D**) Drugs that depress respiratory drive should be avoided in the patient with myxedema coma because they compound the pre-existing respiratory depression. It is appropriate to administer exogenous thyroid hormone replacements, such as I.V. thyroxine. Steroids such as hydrocortisone help the patient respond to stress and are appropriate for those patients with coexistent adrenal insufficiency. Maintenance fluid replacement, such as $D_5\frac{1}{2}NS$, is appropriate.

50. (**A**) Positive response to therapy includes increase in body temperature, decrease in body weight, and reduction in nonpitting edema. Patients in myxedema coma are commonly in respiratory acidosis, characterized by a low pH and high Pa_{CO_2}. If the patient is put on ventilatory support, the Pa_{CO_2} should fall and the pH should rise.

51. (**C**) In planning for patients with chronic thyroid dysfunction, it is important to initiate teaching that will allow the patient and/or family to provide the appropriate care at home. These patients should be allowed to perform activities of daily living within their capabilities. Restricting visitors and providing constant environmental stimulation may be deleterious to the stable patient in the rehabilitation phase.

62. On admission, a patient was noted to have regular respirations of increased rate and depth. Which respiratory pattern does this finding describe?

    A. Kussmaul's respirations.
    B. Cheyne-Stokes respirations.
    C. Biot's respirations.
    D. Paradoxical respirations.

63. Dehydration in DKA results primarily from

    A. ADH deficiency.
    B. Decreased medullary blood flow.
    C. Osmotic diuresis.
    D. Diminished oral intake.

64. Signs of DKA the nurse should recognize include

    A. Cool, clammy skin.
    B. Presence of Babinski reflex.
    C. Shallow, rapid respirations.
    D. Excessive thirst.

65. A female patient admitted with a diagnosis of DKA is very lethargic but arousable. Her lips are dry, and her skin is warm and dry. Blood pressure is 110/60, serum glucose 700 mg/dl, and pH 7.26. A prudent nurse would question which of the following orders?

    A. One amp of sodium bicarbonate I.V. push.
    B. One liter of 0.45% saline over 1 hour.
    C. 20 U. of regular insulin I.V. push.
    D. 10 U. regular insulin I.V. per hour.

66. Which of the following is a feature of hyperglycemic, hyperosmolar, nonketotic coma (HHNK) that differentiates it from diabetic ketoacidosis?

    A. Rapidity of onset.
    B. Alterations in osmolarity.
    C. Absence of lipolysis.
    D. Precipitation by stress.

Answers to Questions from page 118

52. (**B**) Parathormone, which is normally secreted by the parathyroid glands, causes alterations in calcium and phosphate. Parathormone increases calcium ion concentation by increasing bone resorption, stimulating reabsorption of calcium in the renal tubules, and enhancing calcium absorption in the intestines through increased renal synthesis of 1,25-dihydroxycholecalciferol from vitamin D. While serum calcium ion concentration rises, serum phosphate concentration drops. The drop is accomplished by the effect of parathormone on the kidneys—diminished reabsorption of phosphate in the renal tubules.

53. (**C**) In primary adrenal insufficiency, generally both glucocorticoids and mineralocorticoids are deficient. In secondary adrenal insufficiency, such as that caused by abrupt withdrawal of corticosteroid therapy, there is not usually a significant effect on mineralocorticoids. Adrenocorticotropic hormone (ACTH) is secreted by the anterior pituitary and stimulates cortisol release from the adrenal cortex. Cortisol is a glucocorticoid with negative feedback effects that regulate the release of ACTH. In primary adrenal insufficiency, cortisol would not be present in sufficient amounts to inhibit the secretion of ACTH. Therefore, excessive secretion of ACTH would exist.

54. (**A**) Hyperpigmentation is usually present in primary adrenal insufficiency but not in secondary adrenal insufficiency. Its presence is thought to be related to elevated ACTH and related peptide levels. Vomiting, muscle weakness, and abdominal pain can be associated with both primary and secondary adrenal insufficiency.

55. (**B**) With decreased aldosterone and cortisol levels, sodium, chloride, and water are excreted in the urine. Potassium is reabsorbed in exchange for the excreted sodium, and the patient develops hyperkalemia, hyponatremia, hypochloremia, and hypovolemia.

67. One finding *inconsistent* with HHNK is

    A. Tachypnea.
    B. Weight gain.
    C. Polyuria.
    D. Polydipsia.

68. By calculating with the following equation

    $$2(Na^+[mEq]) + \frac{blood\ sugar\ (mg/dl)}{18} + \frac{BUN\ (mg/dl)}{3}$$

    the nurse may obtain an estimate of

    A. Anion gap.
    B. GFR.
    C. Serum osmolality.
    D. Electrolyte excretion.

69. Laboratory findings consistent with HHNK include

    A. Presence of ketones.
    B. High urine pH.
    C. Glycosuria.
    D. Hypoglycemia.

70. Which of the following statements concerning HHNK is true?

    A. It occurs primarily in adolescents.
    B. It may be precipitated by drug therapy.
    C. It is associated with juvenile-onset diabetes.
    D. Remissions and exacerbations are common.

71. The primary organ system in maintenance of glucose homeostasis is the

    A. Liver.
    B. Adrenal glands.
    C. Kidney.
    D. Pancreas.

Answers to Questions from page 119

56. (**B**) During adrenal crisis, the patient should be assisted with all activities of daily living. Controlling the environment and providing for adequate rest is essential; therefore, family visits must be monitored. Glucocorticoid preparations are essential during adrenal crisis. The patient should be placed on a high-sodium, low-potassium diet.

57. (**B**) DKA results from an inadequate amount of insulin. This deficiency causes a diminished utilization of available carbohydrate. Metabolic alterations occur in an attempt to provide needed cell energy.

58. (**B**) Decreased tissue glucose stimulates gluconeogenesis in the liver. *Gluconeogenesis* is the formation of glucose from non-carbohydrate sources, primarily amino acids. The amino acids come from body muscles. In addition to amino acids, glucose is synthesized from lactate, glycerol, and pyruvate in gluconeogenesis. The conversion of glycogen to glucose is *glycogenolysis*.

59. (**D**) In diabetic ketoacidosis or starvation, the oxidation of fatty acids provides primary energy for gluconeogenesis.

60. (**A**) In hyperglycemia, administration of insulin serves to lower the plasma glucose, primarily by inhibiting hepatic release of glucose. Availability of glucose facilitates the transport of glucose and potassium across the cell membrane. The result is a lowering of serum levels and a rise in cellular levels of both glucose and potassium. Insulin also aids in correcting the acidosis by inhibiting ketone production.

61. (**C**) DKA may be triggered by conditions that result in increased insulin needs. Exposure to physical or emotional stress, especially infection, as well as to some medications increases insulin requirements. Exercise and weight reduction may decrease insulin requirements. Compliance with prescribed therapy should be investigated when a previously diagnosed diabetic presents with DKA.

72. A patient is given 30 U. of NPH insulin at 6 A.M. Hypoglycemia related to this injection would be most likely to occur at

    A. 8 A.M.
    B. 12 noon.
    C. 4 P.M.
    D. 8 P.M.

73. Signs and symptoms of hypoglycemia may include all *except*

    A. Nightmares.
    B. Polyuria.
    C. Diaphoresis.
    D. Headache.

Answers to Questions from page 120

62. (**A**) Kussmaul's respirations, as described above, is a compensatory response associated with diabetic acidosis and renal disorders. It occurs in response to stimulation of the respiratory center by a drop in pH.

63. (**C**) Osmotic diuresis occurs in DKA when the filtered load of glucose exceeds the reabsorptive capacity of the renal tubules. Glucose remaining in the tubules exerts an osmotic effect, resulting in fluid loss.

64. (**D**) Some of the signs associated with DKA include fruity-smelling breath, dry skin and mucous membranes, polyuria, polydipsia, and Kussmaul's respirations. The other symptoms listed are associated with hypoglycemia.

65. (**A**) Fluid replacement is instituted immediately upon diagnosis of DKA. Rapidity of fluid administration is based on evaluation of volume status. Replacement likely will be accomplished with a saline solution initially, followed by a glucose solution. Sodium bicarbonate is not generally administered unless the pH is 7.0 or less. Administration of bicarbonate in DKA may cause respiratory distress. Rapid correction of pH causes CO_2 to be removed from the cell in exchange for potassium. CO_2 diffuses across the blood-brain barrier more rapidly than bicarbonate. CSF acidosis and respiratory depression may result. Insulin therapy is initiated with regular insulin, by either constant infusion or periodic small I.V. push doses. Insulin may also be given subcutaneously or intramuscularly.

66. (**C**) Both DKA and HHNK are slow in onset, are accompanied by altered serum osmolarity, and may be precipitated by stress. Lipolysis, which is present in DKA, is not seen in HHNK.

74. Symptoms that may suggest hypoglycemia in infants include

   A. High-pitched cry.
   B. Hiccoughs.
   C. Depressed fontanel.
   D. Presence of Babinski reflex.

75. Emergency management of severe hypoglycemia begins with

   A. Normal saline fluid replacement.
   B. Encouragement of oral fluids.
   C. Supplemental oxygen.
   D. Administration of $D_{50}W$ bolus.

Answers to Questions from page 121

67. (**B**) HHNK is generally associated with dry skin and mucous membranes, altered LOC, tachycardia, shallow rapid respirations, polyuria, polydipsia, and weight loss. Seizures may also occur.

68. (**C**) This formula may be used to estimate serum osmolality. The normal range is 275–295 mOsm/kg body weight. Increased osmolality (greater than 330 mOsm/kg) is seen in HHNK.

69. (**C**) As in DKA, glycosuria is seen in HHNK. Serum glucose is elevated, possibly as high as 2800 mg/dl in HHNK. Absence of ketones in urine is seen in HHNK.

70. (**B**) HHNK occurs primarily in people over 60 years of age. It may occur in people with no history of diabetes. Factors possibly contributing to its development include some drugs (such as Dilantin), high-dose thiazide diuretics, glucocorticoids, hyperosmolar dialysates, or hyperalimentation.

71. (**A**) The liver is the primary organ for supplying blood glucose. Hepatic mechanisms for maintaining blood glucose are glycogenolysis (breakdown of glycogen) and gluconeogenesis (formation of glucose).

| Answers to Questions from page 122 | Answers to Questions from page 123 |

72. **(C)** Action of NPH insulin peaks at 8–12 hours and lasts about 24 hours.

73. **(B)** Polyuria is seen with *hyper*glycemia. A wide range of CNS symptoms may be seen with hypoglycemia, ranging from anxiety to coma.

74. **(A)** Hypoglycemia in infants may be suggested by high-pitched cry, lethargy, apnea, tachycardia, and seizures.

75. **(D)** The initial emergency action for severe hypoglycemia is administration of $D_{50}W$.

Bibliography

American Association of Critical-Care Nurses: Core Curriculum for Critical Care Nursing, 3rd ed. W. B. Saunders Co., Philadelphia, 1985.
Presented in a systems approach, utilizing nursing process outline format. Includes salient points relevant to each system. Delineates essential information for a holistic understanding of critical care nursing.

Bates, B.: A Guide to Physical Examination, 3rd ed. J. B. Lippincott Co., Philadelphia, 1983.
Provides a good description of normal physical findings. Presents physical assessment techniques in a basic, easily understood manner. Provides numerous helpful illustrations.

Beland, I. L.: Clinical Nursing: Pathophysiological and Psychosocial Approaches, 4th ed. Macmillan Co., New York, 1981.
Addresses basic pathophysiology of a wide variety of disorders in an easily understood manner. Utilizes holistic approach.

Brunner, L. S., and Suddarth, D. S.: The Lippincott Manual of Nursing Practice, 3rd ed. J. B. Lippincott Co., Philadelphia, 1982.
Content is presented in numerical format and relates to various procedures and disease states. Includes nursing management and goals but is limited in medical management. Critical information is printed throughout text in colored "nursing alert" boxes.

Dillon, R. S.: Handbook of Endocrinology: Diagnosis and Management of Endocrine and Metabolic Disorders, 2nd ed. Lea & Febiger, Philadelphia, 1980.
Deals with endocrine disorders by groups. Explains normal function and then discusses pathophysiology, symptomatology, and management of related abnormalities. Presents complex information in easily understood manner.

Fletcher, B. J.: Quick Reference to Critical Care Nursing. J. B. Lippincott Co., Philadelphia, 1983.
Deals with a wide variety of critical care topics. For each topic, provides brief overview, causes, clinical manifestations, and diagnostic tests, as well as pertinent nursing responsibilities. Nursing measures helpful in prevention of each disorder are also listed.

Ganong, W. F.: Review of Medical Physiology, 11th ed. Lange Medical Publications, Los Altos, 1983.
A concise advanced human physiology text that also includes brief reviews of related anatomy throughout. Includes limited symptomatology of some physiologic disorders.

Guyton, A. C.: Basic Human Physiology: Normal Function and Mechanisms of Disease. W. B. Saunders Co., Philadelphia, 1977.
Readily understood reference for human physiology. Numerous illustrations and tables enhance content.

Jubiz, W.: Endocrinology: A Logical Approach for Clinicians. McGraw-Hill Book Co., New York, 1979.
Logical, concise, and easy to follow. Tables and diagrams are helpful. Content is somewhat abbreviated but is easily understood.

Kinney, M. R., Dear, C. B., Packa, D. R., and Voorman, D. M. (eds.): AACN's Clinical Reference for Critical Care Nursing. McGraw-Hill Book Co., New York, 1981.
A very comprehensive text for critical care nurses. Separate chapters deal with physiology and pathophysiology of body systems.

Larson, E. L., and Vazquez, M. (eds.): Critical Care Nursing. W. B. Saunders Co., Philadelphia, 1983.
An excellent quick reference for critical care nurses. Addresses wide variety of clinical disorders, including an overview of the disorder, pertinent assessment, and priorities of nursing management. Useful appendices for quick reference.

Mazzaferri, E. L. (ed.): Endocrinology: A Review of Clinical Endocrinology, 2nd ed. Medical Examination Publishing Co., U.S.A., 1980.
A comprehensive text that includes some descriptions of endocrine physiology and pathophysiology. Tables and illustrations augment the text. Each chapter is followed by an extensive list of references.

Petersdorf, R. G., Adams, R. D., Braunwald, E., Isselbacher, K. J., and Wilson, J. D. (eds.): Harrison's Principles of Internal Medicine, 10th ed. McGraw-Hill Book Co., New York, 1983.
An excellent resource containing exhaustive content relative to internal medicine. Provides a sound understanding of pathophysiologic basis for diseases as well as appropriate treatment.

Rose, B. D.: Clinical Physiology of Acid-Base and Electrolyte Disorders. McGraw-Hill Book Co., New York, 1977.
Deals in depth with acid-base and electrolyte physiology and pathophysiology. Throughout, clinical situations are given, providing opportunities to apply concepts that are presented. Extremely comprehensive list of references for each chapter.

Thompson, J. M., and Bowers, A. C.: Clinical Manual of Health Assessment. C. V. Mosby Co., St. Louis, 1980.
Comprehensive physical assessment guide that gives descriptions of normals wth explanations and illustrations of deviations from normal. Organized in a systems approach. Each system discussion ends with a post-test for self-assessment.

6 □ THE HEMATOLOGIC SYSTEM

DIANE K. DRESSLER

1. The attraction of neutrophils to a site of infection is known as

   A. Chemotaxis.
   B. Phagocytosis.
   C. Diapedesis.
   D. Leukocytosis.

2. Red blood cell precursors that are useful in assessing RBC production are the

   A. Erythrocytes.
   B. Reticulocytes.
   C. Megakaryocytes.
   D. Myelocytes.

3. The function of fixed histiocytes such as Kupffer cells in the liver is to

   A. Produce antibodies.
   B. Produce antithrombins.
   C. Form scar tissue.
   D. Phagocytize microorganisms.

4. The bone marrow is stimulated to produce red blood cells by

   A. Acidosis.
   B. Alkalosis.
   C. Hypocapnia.
   D. Hypoxemia.

5. The immunoglobulin responsible for a "wheal-flare" type of allergic reaction is

   A. IgM.
   B. IgG.
   C. IgE.
   D. IgD.

6. The serum of a patient with blood type A contains

   A. Anti-A antibodies.
   B. Anti-B antibodies.
   C. Both anti-A and anti-B antibodies.
   D. Neither anti-A nor anti-B antibodies.

7. The type of white blood cell thought to be most important in the body's defense against cancer is the

   A. T-lymphocyte.
   B. Neutrophil.
   C. Monocyte.
   D. Basophil.

8. When a blood vessel is severed, the first physical mechanism of hemostasis to occur is

   A. Vasodilatation.
   B. Fibrin clot formation.
   C. Fibrinolysis.
   D. Vascular spasms.

9. In order to initiate blood clotting, the extrinsic pathway requires the addition of

   A. Antithrombin III.
   B. Thromboplastin.
   C. Activated factor XII.
   D. Fibrin degradation products.

10. An adequate amount of fibrinogen is essential to the clotting process because fibrinogen

    A. Is necessary for fibrinolysis.
    B. Converts prothrombin to thrombin.
    C. Is converted into the fibrin clot.
    D. Converts plasminogen to plasmin.

11. Thrombolytic agents such as streptokinase work by activating the body's own

    A. Fibrinolytic system.
    B. Hemolytic system.
    C. Clotting mechanism.
    D. Immune system.

12. The average adult circulatory system contains _____ L of blood:

    A. 1–2.
    B. 3–4.
    C. 5–6.
    D. 9–10.

13. The lifespan of platelets is normally _____ day(s).

    A. 1.
    B. 3–4.
    C. 9–12.
    D. 21.

14. Most plasma coagulation factors are synthesized in the

   A. Thymus.
   B. Spleen.
   C. Bone marrow.
   D. Liver.

15. Cellular immunity is carried out by

   A. Specific antibodies.
   B. Sensitized lymphocytes (T-cells).
   C. Megakaryocytes.
   D. Eosinophils.

16. The _____ system plays a major role in the prevention of edema.

   A. Complement.
   B. Reticuloendothelial.
   C. Lymphatic.
   D. Hematopoietic.

17. In addition to distributing T- and B-cells, the lymph nodes

   A. Filter bacteria and foreign particles.
   B. Produce neutrophils.
   C. Produce hormones.
   D. Synthesize coagulation factors.

18. Fully differentiated lymphocytes that produce specific antibodies are known as

   A. T-lymphocytes.
   B. Plasma cells.
   C. Erythrocytes.
   D. Monocytes.

19. Rejection of transplanted organs occurs as a function of

   A. Interferon.
   B. Segmented neutrophils.
   C. Cellular immunity.
   D. Humoral immunity.

20. Physiologic protection against excessive clotting and thrombosis depends in part on the presence of adequate amounts of

   A. Platelets.
   B. Factor V.
   C. Calcium.
   D. Antithrombin III.

Answers to Questions from page 127

1. (**A**) *Chemotaxis* refers to the ability to attract white blood cells. *Phagocytosis* is the engulfing of bacteria by WBCs. *Diapedesis* is the process by which WBCs pass through vessel walls. *Leukocytosis* is a rise in WBC count.

2. (**B**) RBC precursors are reticulocytes. Erythrocytes are mature RBCs. Megakaryocytes are platelet precursors. Myelocytes are WBC precursors.

3. (**D**) Fixed histiocytes phagocytize microorganisms and other particles. Antibodies are produced by plasma cells. Antithrombins are produced by other parts of the liver. Scar tissue is formed by fibroblasts.

4. (**D**) Hypoxemia, or low blood oxygen level, is known to stimulate RBC production.

5. (**C**) IgE immunoglobulins induce histamine release, which mediates the inflammatory reaction. IgM and IgG are most influential against bacteria. IgD is believed to activate B-cells to plasma cells.

6. (**B**) The type of antibodies that develop in the serum depends on which antigen is *not* present; thus, people with type A blood will develop anti-B antibodies.

21. Naturally occurring protein that interferes with viral growth is known as

    A. Complement.
    B. Interferon.
    C. Migration inhibiting factor (MIF).
    D. Transfer factor.

22. One of the most important parts of a hematologic assessment is evaluation of

    A. Cardiac function.
    B. Vital signs.
    C. Patient and family history.
    D. Cognitive function.

23. Hemolytic anemia is *more likely* to develop in patients with a history of

    A. Prosthetic heart valve implantation.
    B. Total hip replacement.
    C. Coronary artery bypass grafting.
    D. Abdominal aneurysm repair.

24. The first clinical sign of platelet dysfunction is often

    A. Hematuria.
    B. Petechiae.
    C. Hemorrhage.
    D. Hematoma.

25. Physical signs of hemolytic anemia often include

    A. Pallor and lymphadenopathy.
    B. Pallor and muscle atrophy.
    C. Jaundice and lymphadenopathy.
    D. Jaundice and splenomegaly.

26. A laboratory report of leukocyte "shift to the left" with the appearance of "band" neutrophils may suggest the presence of a(n)

    A. Neutropenia.
    B. Acute infection.
    C. Anemia.
    D. Thrombocytopenia.

27. Your patient's preoperative lab work shows a platelet count of 25,000/mm^3. The following nursing action is indicated:

    A. Request an order to administer vitamin K.
    B. Start an I.V. immediately.
    C. Notify the surgeon of this lab result.
    D. No action is necessary, since this is a normal platelet count.

Answers to Questions from page 128

7. (**A**) T-lymphocytes are involved in defense against cancer. Neutrophils and monocytes defend against microorganisms. Basophils are active in allergic responses and chronic inflammation.

8. (**D**) Spasm of the vessel occurs first; it decreases blood loss while the processes of platelet plugging and blood clotting occur. Fibrinolysis dissolves clots.

9. (**B**) Injured tissues release thromboplastin, which is necessary to activate the extrinsic pathway. Antithrombin III inactivates thrombin. Factor XII is involved in activating the intrinsic pathway. Fibrin degradation products result from fibrinolysis.

10. (**C**) Fibrinogen is converted into the fibrin strands that form the fibrin clot. Fibrinolysis dissolves the clot. Activated factor X converts prothrombin to thrombin. Plasminogen is converted to plasmin by plasminogen activators.

11. (**A**) The fibrinolytic system is activated, lysing clots and recanalizing the vessel. Thrombolytic agents do not act by causing hemolysis, clotting, or immune reactions.

12. (**C**) The normal blood volume is 5–6 L.

13. (**C**) Platelets' normal lifespan is 9–12 days.

28. For patients receiving Coumadin, a pro-thrombin time of 50 seconds (control 12 seconds) would be interpreted as

    A. Slightly excessive anticoagulation.
    B. Insufficient anticoagulation.
    C. Optimal anticoagulation.
    D. A value that should be reported immediately.

29. Diagnostic studies done to distinguish between the various types of anemia would include

    A. BUN and creatinine.
    B. Peripheral blood smear and bone marrow biopsy.
    C. Erythrocyte sedimentation rate (ESR) and WBC.
    D. Long-bone x-rays.

30. A single aspirin may cause abnormalities in platelet function for as long as _____ day(s).

    A. 1.
    B. 2.
    C. 5.
    D. 9–12.

31. During massive transfusion therapy, the ECG should be observed for changes indicative of

    A. First-degree heart block.
    B. Junctional tachycardia.
    C. Hyperkalemia.
    D. Hypokalemia.

32. Nursing care of the bleeding patient should generally include

    A. Avoidance of iced water.
    B. Bedrest.
    C. Progression of activity as tolerated.
    D. Close monitoring of body temperature.

33. Osteoporosis is commonly seen in advanced stages of

    A. Chronic lymphocytic leukemia.
    B. Lymphosarcoma.
    C. Hodgkin's disease.
    D. Multiple myeloma.

Answers to Questions from page 129

14. (**D**) The liver produces most coagulation factors, including prothrombin, fibrinogen, and factors V, VII, IX, and X.

15. (**B**) Cellular immunity involves the release of sensitized lymphocytes to destroy antigens. Humoral immunity is mediated by antibodies. Megakaryocytes are platelet precursors. Eosinophils are active in allergic reactions.

16. (**C**) The lymphatic system returns interstitial fluid to the heart, thereby preventing edema. The complement system is involved in immune reactions. The reticuloendothelial and hematopoietic systems do not directly prevent edema.

17. (**A**) The lymph nodes filter bacteria and particulate matter. Neutrophils are produced in the bone marrow. Hormones are produced in other organs, such as the pituitary gland and adrenal gland. Most coagulation factors are produced in the liver.

18. (**B**) Plasma cells are sensitized B-cells that produce specific antibodies. T-lymphocytes function in cellular immunity. Erythrocytes carry oxygen, and monocytes function in phagocytosis of microorganisms and particulate matter.

19. (**C**) Allograft rejection is mediated by cellular immunity (T-cells). Interferon suppresses viral growth. Segmented neutrophils are involved in the defense against microorganisms.

20. (**D**) Antithrombin III inactivates thrombin and prevents thrombosis. The other factors listed are procoagulants.

34. Prior to an operation or invasive procedure, nursing responsibilities include checking the patient's medication profile for

    A. Calcium antagonists.
    B. Antihypertensives.
    C. Anticoagulants.
    D. Antibiotics.

35. In managing the care of patients with bleeding disorders, an important protective function of the nurse is to

    A. Provide adequate hydration.
    B. Minimize invasive procedures.
    C. Observe for dysrhythmias.
    D. Administer blood components.

36. When a transfusion reaction is suspected, the first action generally taken is to

    A. Stop the blood or blood component infusion.
    B. Slow the rate of blood or blood component infusion.
    C. Notify the blood bank.
    D. Notify the physician.

37. A unit of fresh frozen plasma should be administered

    A. As rapidly as tolerated.
    B. Over about 1 hour.
    C. Over about 2 hours.
    D. Over about 4 hours.

38. The blood component that is generally stored at room temperature is

    A. Cryoprecipitate.
    B. Red cell mass.
    C. Platelet concentrate.
    D. Whole blood.

39. The clotting factors supplied by cryoprecipitate are

    A. Factors V and VII.
    B. Fibrinogen and factor VIII.
    C. Factors IX and X.
    D. Prothrombin and calcium.

40. Blood volume expansion in a hypovolemic patient would be achieved most effectively by the administration of

    A. Platelet concentrate.
    B. Granulocyte concentrate.
    C. Frozen red cells.
    D. Plasma protein fraction.

Answers to Questions from page 130

21. (**B**) Interferon suppresses viral growth. Complement enhances the function of antibodies. MIF prevents the movement of macrophages. Transfer factor enables immune responses to be transferred from sensitized individuals to nonsensitized individuals.

22. (**C**) Although all of these aspects might be included, a patient or family history of hematologic abnormalities is extremely important in patient assessment.

23. (**A**) Prosthetic heart valve malfunction or paravalvular leaking can result in hemolytic anemia.

24. (**B**) Since platelets normally plug small tears in capillaries, petechiae occur as early signs of thrombocytopenia and platelet dysfunction.

25. (**D**) Jaundice and splenomegaly occur from the excessive destruction of RBCs, which results in elevated bilirubin levels and accumulation of defective cells in the spleen and liver.

26. (**B**) An increase in immature "band" neutrophils is a characteristic response to acute infection.

27. (**C**) A normal platelet count is 150,000 to 400,000/mm^3. This patient's platelet count is not adequate for hemostasis.

41. The mean incubation time for transfusion-related hepatitis is

    A. 5 days.
    B. 50 days.
    C. 1 year.
    D. 2 years.

42. When preparing a patient for a bone marrow biopsy, the nurse should explain that the biopsy site is usually the

    A. Fifth rib.
    B. Posterior iliac crest.
    C. Anterior tibia.
    D. Distal humerus.

43. The basic defect in sickle cell anemia is

    A. Lack of sufficient globin molecules.
    B. Red cell membrane abnormalities.
    C. Deficient amount of the enzyme G6PD.
    D. Lack of hemoglobin A (normal hemoglobin).

44. For patients with sickle cell anemia, a sickle cell crisis might be precipitated by an environment with

    A. Excessive humidity.
    B. Extreme dryness.
    C. High altitude.
    D. High temperature.

45. In managing the care of a patient in sickle cell crisis, it is important that the nurse provide enough

    A. Oxygen and fluids.
    B. Protein and calories.
    C. Activity and exercise.
    D. Chemotherapy.

46. A stable adult patient with anemia would most likely be transfused when the

    A. Hemoglobin drops to 10 gm/dl.
    B. Hematocrit drops to 30%.
    C. Patient develops signs and symptoms such as hypotension.
    D. Platelet count drops to 50,000/mm³.

47. Teaching the patient with pernicious anemia includes making sure he or she understands the lifelong necessity of

    A. Periodic blood transfusions.
    B. Periodic platelet transfusions.
    C. Vitamin K injections.
    D. Vitamin B$_{12}$ injections.

Answers to Questions from page 131

28. **(D)** This patient is at risk for hemorrhage due to excessive anticoagulation. Optimal anticoagulation with Coumadin is 1½ to 2 times the control value, in this case 18 to 24 seconds.

29. **(B)** The blood smear and bone marrow biopsy often reveal diagnostic indicators of specific anemias. BUN and creatinine are indices of renal function. ESR and WBC change in inflammation. Long-bone x-rays may be included in the diagnosis of leukemia.

30. **(D)** Aspirin inhibits platelet function for the life of the platelet (9–12 days).

31. **(C)** Hyperkalemia—indicated by large peaked T waves, an acute injury pattern, and bradycardia—may result from massive transfusion. Stored blood has a high serum potassium level, because the red cell lysis associated with transfusion causes intracellular potassium ions to be released into the plasma.

32. **(B)** Bedrest is recommended during bleeding episodes. Iced water may be employed to stop bleeding. Body temperature is not a major parameter affected by bleeding.

33. **(D)** In multiple myeloma, areas of bone are destroyed in the skull, vertebrae, and ribs. Lytic bone lesions are much less common in the other diseases listed.

48. A cardiac patient with severe anemia may experience

    A. Angina.
    B. Hemorrhage.
    C. Pericarditis.
    D. Hypertension.

49. Patients with anemia should know that foods rich in iron include

    A. Bananas, orange juice, and broth.
    B. Liver, red meat, and kidney beans.
    C. Canned vegetables, bacon, and hot dogs.
    D. Potato chips, potatoes, and citrus fruit.

50. 2 U. of red cell mass would provide your patient with the same oxygen-carrying capacity as _____U. of whole blood.

    A. 1.
    B. 2.
    C. 3.
    D. 4.

51. A common complication of polycythemia vera is

    A. Recurrent urinary tract infection.
    B. Venous thrombosis.
    C. Electrolyte imbalance.
    D. Renal lithiasis.

52. The CBC of a patient with polycythemia vera will show an elevated hemoglobin plus

    A. Decreased WBCs and platelets.
    B. Presence of sickled RBCs.
    C. Increased WBCs and platelets.
    D. Abnormal leukocytes.

53. Pharmacologic treatment for polycythemia vera may include

    A. Antihypertensive drugs.
    B. Antibiotics.
    C. Steroids.
    D. Myelosuppressive drugs.

54. In assessing a patient with suspected anaphylaxis, it would be particularly important to listen to

    A. Bowel tones.
    B. Heart sounds.
    C. Breath sounds.
    D. Carotid bruits.

Answers to Questions from page 132

34. **(C)** The physician must be informed if the patient has been receiving anticoagulants, including platelet inhibitors such as aspirin.

35. **(B)** Although the nurse may carry out any of these functions, the important protective function is to minimize or prevent invasive procedures, which may precipitate bleeding episodes.

36. **(A)** First, the blood should be stopped if a reaction is suspected, and then the appropriate others should be notified.

37. **(A)** Fresh frozen plasma is administered as rapidly as tolerated so that it is infused before factors become inactive. Some coagulation factors have a metabolic half-life of only a few hours.

38. **(C)** Platelet concentrate is generally stored at room temperature. The other components are refrigerated or frozen.

39. **(B)** Cryoprecipitate is given specifically to replace fibrinogen and factor VIII (antihemophilic factor). Fresh frozen plasma would be administered if all clotting factors were needed.

40. **(D)** Plasma protein fraction is the most effective of these volume expanders. The addition of protein to the vascular compartment raises its oncotic pressure, thereby drawing interstitial fluid into the vascular compartment and expanding circulating blood volume. The other components could also provide volume expansion but more likely would be given for specific blood element deficiencies.

55. Emergency treatment of anaphylaxis usually begins with the administration of

    A. Epinephrine.
    B. Sodium bicarbonate.
    C. Digoxin.
    D. Xylocaine.

56. In a patient with decreased white blood cells, the most important sign of infection to watch for is

    A. Pulmonary infiltrates.
    B. Fever.
    C. Redness and swelling.
    D. Pus formation.

57. Patients with neutropenia need routine assessment of the oral mucosa for

    A. Herpes infection.
    B. Areas of hemorrhage.
    C. Gingivitis.
    D. Candidiasis.

58. A metabolic abnormality that commonly occurs in leukemia is

    A. Hyperglycemia.
    B. Hyperuricemia.
    C. Hypoglycemia.
    D. Hypocalcemia.

59. A patient with leukemia who is in "partial remission" still has evidence of the disease in the

    A. Bone marrow.
    B. Peripheral blood.
    C. Spleen.
    D. Liver.

60. A common physical finding in both acute and chronic lymphocytic leukemia is

    A. Leg ulcers.
    B. Massive splenomegaly.
    C. Severe bone pain.
    D. Lymphadenopathy.

61. For a patient with leukemia, an important daily nursing action would be to check the most recent

    A. Urinalysis results.
    B. Electrocardiogram.
    C. CBC.
    D. Serum electrolyte values.

Answers to Questions from page 133

41. **(B)** The mean incubation time, or average time before clinical signs of hepatitis appear, is 50 days.

42. **(B)** The posterior iliac crest is most commonly used, but occasionally the sternum or anterior iliac crest is used.

43. **(D)** In sickle cell anemia, red cells lack hemoglobin A and instead contain hemoglobin S.

44. **(C)** High altitude can precipitate sickle cell crisis, because hypoxia leads to sickling.

45. **(A)** Oxygen prevents further hypoxia and sickling, and fluids decrease blood viscosity and improve circulation.

46. **(C)** Transfusions are generally given when the patient becomes symptomatic.

47. **(D)** Vitamin B_{12} injections are administered monthly to patients with pernicious anemia because such patients lack the intrinsic factor necessary to absorb the vitamin through the GI tract. Blood and platelet transfusions would not normally be necessary. Vitamin K is not indicated for anemia.

62. It is unlikely that a person more than 20 years old will acquire

   A. Hodgkin's disease.
   B. Acute lymphoblastic leukemia.
   C. Chronic lymphoblastic leukemia.
   D. Multiple myeloma.

63. In chronic leukemia, a "blastic crisis"

   A. Stimulates platelet production.
   B. Stimulates production of mature neutrophils.
   C. Increases the chance of remission.
   D. Changes chronic leukemia to acute leukemia.

64. During the administration of intravenous antileukemic drugs such as vincristine and daunorubicin, great care is taken to avoid

   A. Infiltration of the chemotherapeutic agent.
   B. Diluting the medication.
   C. Interrupting the patient's meals.
   D. Interrupting the patient's sleep.

65. Patients with leukemia are more likely to develop neurologic problems because of

   A. Cerebral emboli.
   B. Psychological depression.
   C. Central nervous system metastasis.
   D. Head trauma.

66. Multiple myeloma is a neoplastic disorder of the

   A. Spleen.
   B. Liver.
   C. Plasma cells.
   D. T-lymphocytes.

67. Priorities of nursing care in the patient with multiple myeloma include

   A. Fluid restriction and bedrest.
   B. Ambulation and adequate hydration.
   C. Administration of oxygen and IPPB.
   D. A diet high in iron.

Answers to Questions from page 134

48. **(A)** Severe anemia is likely to precipitate angina because of the increased demands that anemia places on the heart (increased heart rate and contractility) and the heart's inability to meet these demands.

49. **(B)** Liver, red meat, and kidney beans, as well as whole wheat bread, spinach, egg yolk, raisins, and apricots, are high in iron.

50. **(B)** Each unit of red cell mass has the same oxygen-carrying capacity as one unit of whole blood.

51. **(B)** Venous thrombosis commonly results from the increased blood viscosity associated with polycythemia vera.

52. **(C)** WBCs and platelets are also elevated in polycythemia vera because the disorder is actually a panmyelosis belonging to the myeloproliferative disorders. Sickled cells are seen in sickle cell anemia. Abnormal leukocytes are seen in leukemia.

53. **(D)** Chemotherapy with myelosuppressive drugs such as chlorambucil, cyclophosphamide, and melphalan may be used along with phlebotomy, hydration, and irradiation.

54. **(C)** Auscultation of breath sounds to detect bronchospasm, a common clinical sign of anaphylaxis, would be most important.

68. Stages I and II of Hodgkin's disease are most commonly treated with

    A. Surgery.
    B. Chemotherapy.
    C. Radiation.
    D. Immune therapy.

69. The staging procedure in Hodgkin's disease may include a(n)

    A. Feeding gastrostomy.
    B. Cystoscopy.
    C. Carotid arteriography.
    D. Exploratory laparotomy.

70. Skin care for the patient receiving radiation therapy should include

    A. Daily fresh air and sun exposure.
    B. Bathing of radiated areas with tepid water.
    C. Backrubs with alcohol.
    D. Vigorous washing of radiotherapy markings.

71. Classic hemophilia (hemophilia A) is an inherited bleeding disorder characterized by a deficiency of

    A. Factor VIII.
    B. Factor VII.
    C. Factor V.
    D. Platelets.

72. In disseminated intravascular coagulation (DIC), the blood becomes depleted in

    A. Calcium.
    B. Many clotting factors, including platelets.
    C. Albumin.
    D. Essential hormones.

73. Blood coagulation study results indicative of DIC include

    A. Lack of fibrin monomers and schistocytes.
    B. Factor V and VIII levels above 80%.
    C. Normal prothrombin time (PT) and an elevated partial thromboplastin time (PTT).
    D. Decrease in platelets and the presence of fibrinolysis.

Answers to Questions from page 135

55. (**A**) Epinephrine is administered first, either subcutaneously, I.M., or I.V., to reverse the bronchospasm and vasodilation. Other emergency medications may be indicated later.

56. (**B**) Fever may be the only clinical manifestation of infection. Other signs of infection may not occur in neutropenia because they depend on WBC levels.

57. (**D**) Candidiasis, a fungal infection, occurs frequently in neutropenia.

58. (**B**) Hyperuricemia occurs in leukemia from cellular proliferation and necrosis and from the accumulation of cellular waste products secondary to therapy.

59. (**A**) Partial remission indicates there is still evidence of the disease in the bone marrow. In complete remission, there is no evidence of disease in the peripheral blood or bone marrow.

60. (**D**) Lymphadenopathy occurs as lymphocytes accumulate in the lymph nodes. Leg ulcers are common in sickle cell anemia. Massive splenomegaly and bone pain are associated with myelocytic leukemia.

61. (**C**) It would be most important to check the CBC to determine the severity of anemia, neutropenia, and thrombocytopenia.

74. Pain intervention for the bleeding patient may be difficult because

    A. The patient may not respond to narcotics.
    B. The patient may refuse medication.
    C. Analgesics may contribute to hypertension.
    D. Analgesics may contribute to hypotension.

Answers to Questions from page 136

62. (**B**) Peak incidence of acute lymphoblastic leukemia is 1 to 5 years of age; it seldom occurs after 20. The other diseases commonly occur in individuals over 20 years of age.

63. (**D**) A "blastic crisis" changes chronic leukemia to acute leukemia; following such a crisis, only palliative therapy is provided.

64. (**A**) Infiltration is carefully avoided because it can lead to extravasation and severe tissue damage.

65. (**C**) In patients with leukemia, neurologic complaints are often due to central nervous system metastasis.

66. (**C**) Multiple myeloma is characterized by malignant proliferation of the plasma cells.

67. (**B**) In order to minimize osteoporosis and calcium overload, activity and fluid intake are encouraged. Respiratory therapy and a diet high in iron might be indicated in any hematologic disorder and would not have a particular priority in multiple myeloma.

75. Early clinical manifestations of DIC often include

    A. Petechiae and pruritis.
    B. Oozing of blood from incisions or puncture sites.
    C. Fever and shaking chills.
    D. Renal failure.

Answers to Questions from page 137

68. **(C)** Radiation is used to treat the early stages of Hodgkin's disease. Radiation and/or chemotherapy may be used for later stages. Surgery and immune therapy would not be commonly used as treatment.

69. **(D)** Exploratory laparotomy is often part of the staging procedure for Hodgkin's disease.

70. **(B)** Gentle bathing of radiated areas with tepid water is indicated. The other actions would be contraindicated, because sun exposure would increase skin reactions, topical agents such as alcohol could further irritate skin, and radiotherapy markings must be left intact.

71. **(A)** A deficiency of factor VIII (antihemophilic factor) results in classic hemophilia. Deficiencies of the other factors might result in other bleeding problems, such as postoperative bleeding.

72. **(B)** DIC leads to depletion of many clotting factors, which are consumed as clots form in the microcirculation.

73. **(D)** Platelets are decreased and fibrinolysis is present in DIC. Other findings may include the presence of fibrin monomers and schistocytes, low levels of factor V and VIII, and abnormal PT and PTT.

74. (**D**) Administration of analgesics I.M. or I.V. to a patient who is hypovolemic may lead to severe hypotension.

75. (**B**) DIC often initially manifests as generalized oozing. Petechiae may or may not develop, and renal failure may occur late in the syndrome. Fever and shaking chills would generally not occur as a result of DIC.

Bibliography

Coleman, R. W., Hirsh, J., Marder, V. J., and Saltzman, E. W.: Hemostasis and Thrombosis. J. B. Lippincott Co., Philadelphia, 1982.
Contains extensive coverage of virtually all clinically important coagulation problems. Major sections on congenital hemorrhagic disorders, the physiology of clotting, platelet production and destruction, platelet dysfunction, acquired coagulation disorders, and thromboembolism.

Erslev, A. J., and Gabuzda, T. G.: Pathophysiology of Blood, 2nd ed. W. B. Saunders Co., Philadelphia, 1979.
Detailed information related to the production of cellular components and plasma coagulation factors. Text is enhanced by photographs and diagrams. Includes brief descriptions of hematologic disorders.

Gunz, F. W., and Henderson, E. S. (eds.): Leukemia. Grune & Stratton, New York, 1983.
Pathophysiology of leukemia is presented through contributions of many experts. A section is devoted to the etiology. Clinical diagnosis, treatment, and medical management are covered extensively.

Guyton, A. C.: Textbook of Medical Physiology, 6th ed. W. B. Saunders Co., Philadelphia, 1981. Chapter 9: "Hemostasis and Blood Coagulation."
A concise and exceptionally clear description of the physical and biochemical events in blood coagulation. Also includes brief descriptions of a few major bleeding and thrombotic conditions.

Hirsh, J., and Brain, E.: Hemostasis and Thrombosis: A Conceptual Approach. Churchill Livingstone, New York, 1979.
Illustrated descriptions of the events in blood coagulation. Major topics include blood coagulation, abnormal hemostasis mechanisms, clinical and laboratory indicators of coagulation disorders, and thrombosis.

Luckman, J., and Sorenson, K. C.: Medical-Surgical Nursing, 2nd ed. W. B. Saunders Co., Philadelphia, 1980. Unit XIV: "Nursing People Experiencing Disturbance of the Blood and Blood Forming Organs."
Summarizes the anatomy and physiology of the hematologic system. Also includes description of the major blood dyscrasias and nursing responsibilities related to the care of affected patients.

Merskey, C.: DIC: Identification and management. Hosp. Pract. *17*: 83–94, 1982.
Describes current thought related to the pathogenesis of DIC. Also includes associated clinical conditions, laboratory indicators, and current medical management.

Rutman, R. C., and Miller, W. V.: Transfusion Therapy: Principles and Procedures. Aspen Systems Corp., Rockville, Maryland, 1981.
Includes information related to processing and distribution of blood and blood components in addition to procedures detailing the administration. Emphasizes nursing implications of transfusion therapy.

Thomson, J. M. (ed.): Blood Coagulation and Haemostasis. Churchill Livingstone, New York, 1980.
Detailed discussion of current studies pertaining to inherited and acquired bleeding disorders. Emphasizes diagnosis and laboratory features.

Williams, W. J., Beutler, E., Erslev, A. J., and Lichtman, M. A.: Hematology. McGraw-Hill Book Co., New York, 1983.
Comprehensive volume covering all aspects of clinical hematology. Presents disorders of blood cells and defects of hemostasis. Descriptions of patient history, clinical manifestations, and laboratory studies are especially helpful.

7 □ THE GASTROINTESTINAL SYSTEM

MAURENE A. HARVEY

1. During deglutition, the airway is protected by

   A. Closing of the hypopharyngeal sphincter.
   B. Opening of the gastrointestinal sphincter.
   C. Contraction of the oropharynx.
   D. Closure of the epiglottis.

2. Gastric mechanical activity during ingestion can be described as a process in which

   A. The goal is rapid gastric emptying.
   B. Liquids are evacuated before solids.
   C. The stomach is very noncompliant.
   D. Chyme is mixed and slowly propelled through the cardiac sphincter.

3. Factors that stimulate gastric emptying include

   A. Emotions such as pain, anxiety, and depression.
   B. A high-fat meal.
   C. Low gastric pH.
   D. Cholinergic agents.

4. Gastric secretion of hydrochloric acid increases in response to

   A. The release of histamine.
   B. Anticholinergic agents.
   C. Cimetidine.
   D. A pH of chyme below 2.0.

5. The mucosal barrier protects the cells lining the stomach by

   A. Secreting the intrinsic factor.
   B. Being permeable to substances such as bile salts.
   C. Limiting pH changes to near neutral levels.
   D. Preventing back-diffusion of HCl into the mucosal cells.

6. An example of the lymphoid cells in the lining of the gastrointestinal tract that are involved in immune defenses is

   A. Peyer's patches.
   B. Brunner's cells.
   C. Lacteals.
   D. Oxyntic cells.

7. Motility of the small intestine

   A. Is constant at a steady rate during fasting states.
   B. Is primarily aboral.
   C. Is only peristaltic.
   D. Consists of single long rostrocaudal waves.

8. An example of an active transport mechanism that is involved in intestinal absorption is

   A. Osmosis of water along concentration gradients.
   B. Fructose diffusion.
   C. Fatty acid diffusion.
   D. Electrolyte absorption.

9. The end products of nutrient digestion, after both intraluminal and intracellular processes in the small intestine are completed, include

   A. Maltose, sucrose, and lactose.
   B. Peptides and proteases.
   C. Fatty acids and glycerol.
   D. Lipids and triglycerides.

10. Motility of the large intestine is increased by

    A. A diet low in residue.
    B. The presence of *Escherichia coli*.
    C. Hypotonic contents.
    D. An increased level of bile salts.

11. Functions of the large intestine include

    A. Production of urea from ammonia.
    B. Absorption of the majority of nutrients.
    C. Potassium and bicarbonate absorption in exchange for sodium and chloride secretion.
    D. Water absorption.

12. An example of a substance that directly affects gastrointestinal function through nerve transmission is

    A. A cholinergic agent.
    B. Gastrin.
    C. Secretin.
    D. Cholecystokinin.

13. A hormone that stimulates the secretory activities of the stomach is

    A. Cholecystokinin.
    B. Secretin.
    C. Gastrin.
    D. Glucagon.

14. The hormone that seems to be the most potent stimulant for bicarbonate production by the pancreas is

    A. Cholecystokinin.
    B. Secretin.
    C. Gastrin.
    D. Vasoactive intestinal peptide.

15. A hormone that acts on liver, fat, and muscle cells to inhibit glucose production is

    A. Insulin.
    B. Glucagon.
    C. Secretin.
    D. Gastrin.

16. Which of the following statements concerning glucagon is *true?*

    A. It is a form of stored carbohydrate.
    B. It is a hormone produced by the beta cells in the pancreas.
    C. It promotes glycogenesis.
    D. It promotes gluconeogenesis.

17. Diagnostic and therapeutic procedures for upper gastrointestinal diseases are most likely to involve cannulation of which arterial system?

    A. Celiac.
    B. Superior mesenteric.
    C. Inferior mesenteric.
    D. Portal.

18. The efferent vessels of the liver are the

    A. Hepatic arteries.
    B. Hepatic veins.
    C. Portal veins.
    D. Hepatic ducts.

| **Answers to Questions from page 143** |

1. (**D**) During deglutition, flow is directed into the esophagus during contraction of the oropharynx by opening of the hypopharyngeal sphincter and closing of alternative pathways. The airway is protected by closure of the epiglottis.

2. (**B**) During ingestion, the stomach relaxes (increases compliance) to act as a reservoir until its contents are mixed, its secretions are released, and the duodenum can accept a bolus of chyme. Chyme is released through the pylorus (into small intestine), and not the cardiac sphincter (into esophagus). Liquids are evacuated earlier than solids.

3. (**D**) Although the effect of emotions on gastric emptying is complex, immobilizing feelings seem to suppress the process. High-fat diets and acidic gastric contents retard motility, whereas cholinergic nervous impulses stimulate it.

4. (**A**) Gastric secretion of hydrochloric acid is increased by histamine (cimetidine blocks it), by cholinergic nervous impulses, and by release of gastrin. Gastrin release is inhibited by acid chyme. The sight, smell, and taste of food stimulate the cholinergic nerves (the cephalic stage).

5. (**D**) The mucus secreted to line the gastric mucosa allows HCl to diffuse into the stomach and therefore create a highly acidic environment. The mucosa prevents diffusion of HCl back into the cells, thereby protecting them. The barrier is permeable, however, to certain other acids, such as bile salts and salicylates, a feature that may lead to damage.

19. Intrinsic sympathetic nerve fibers innervating the gastrointestinal tract

    A. Are primarily contained in the vagus nerve.
    B. Secrete acetylcholine.
    C. Originate from cranial and sacral nerves.
    D. Are found in both the inner and outer walls of the intestine.

20. The acinar secretions of the pancreas

    A. Include the hormones insulin and glucagon.
    B. Are highly acidic solutions and contain many digestive enzymes.
    C. Are suppressed by vagal stimulation.
    D. Are regulated in part by secretin and cholecystokinin.

21. Which of the following substrates is responsible for emulsifying fats in the gastrointestinal tract?

    A. Bile.
    B. Lipase.
    C. Amylase.
    D. Gastrin.

22. Which of the following statements regarding bilirubin is *false*?

    A. Bilirubin production may increase in patients with hemolytic anemia.
    B. Bilirubin is converted from an unconjugated to a conjugated form in the liver.
    C. Conjugated bilirubin is converted to urobilinogen in the kidneys.
    D. The reticuloendothelial system is the primary source of unconjugated bilirubin found in the blood stream.

23. The expected laboratory finding in the jaundiced patient with biliary tract obstruction without associated liver cell damage is

    A. Increased urobilinogen.
    B. Increased total bilirubin with the unconjugated form dominating.
    C. Increased total bilirubin with the conjugated form dominating.
    D. Increased total bilirubin and increased urobilinogen.

6. (**A**) Peyer's patches are made up of lymphocytes residing in the gastrointestinal tract. Brunner's cells secrete mucus. Oxyntic cells secrete hydrochloric acid and intrinsic factor. Lacteals are lymph vessels, not cells.

7. (**B**) The mobility of the small intestine consists of both segmental and peristaltic contractions. It varies greatly even during the fasting state. Although impulses spread in both directions, the overall movement is toward the rectum (aboral) and usually affects only small portions of the small bowel at any one time.

8. (**D**) Water is absorbed primarily via osmosis, which is a passive phenomenon. Fatty acids and fructose similarly follow passive concentration gradients, although fructose requires facilitation. The electrolytes, however, must be actively transported by energy-consuming mechanisms to prevent inappropriate losses.

9. (**C**) Carbohydrate digestion proceeds from polysaccharides to disaccharides (maltose, sucrose, and lactose) to monosaccharides or simple sugars (fructose, glucose, and galactose). Proteins are broken down into amino acids. Fats and triglycerides become fatty acids and glycerol. The end-product stage must be reached before nutrients can be absorbed from intestinal cells into capillaries and lacteals.

10. (**D**) Motility is increased by high-residual diets, hypertonic contents, and bile salts. Bacterial endotoxins can increase motility, but *Escherichia coli* is part of the normal intestinal flora.

11. (**D**) Ammonia is made by intestinal cells from the breakdown of urea. The majority of nutrients are absorbed in the jejunum. Sodium and chloride are absorbed and potassium and bicarbonate are secreted by the large intestine. One of the primary functions of the colon is to reabsorb water.

12. (**A**) Acetylcholine (cholinergic agent) and norepinephrine (adrenergic agent) are primary substances linking nerves across synapses in the gastrointestinal tract. Gastrin and secretin, which are hormones, are secreted into the blood stream and act indirectly. Cholecystokinin, also a hormone, is secreted by nerves but is released into the blood stream.

24. The functions of the Kupffer cells in the liver include

    A. Synthesis of plasma clotting factors.
    B. Synthesis of glucose from fatty acids and amino acids when needed.
    C. Synthesis of glycogen.
    D. Phagocytosis of bacteria.

25. A patient complaining of a dull, diffuse abdominal pain is more likely to have

    A. Cholecystitis.
    B. Appendicitis.
    C. Intestinal obstruction.
    D. Pelvic inflammatory disease.

26. One normal finding during inspection of the abdomen would be

    A. Visibility of engorged superficial veins.
    B. Lower abdominal pulsations.
    C. Visibility of peristalsis.
    D. Movement associated with the ventilatory cycle in men.

27. The sounds most likely to be heard over the abdomen in a patient with early intestinal obstruction are

    A. Intermittent soft gurgling sounds at the rate of approximately 20 per minute.
    B. Loud, high-pitched, tinkling borborygmi.
    C. Hypoactive sounds due to intestinal muscle weakness.
    D. Peritoneal friction rubs.

28. The auscultatory finding most directly related to portal hypertension is a

    A. Succussion splash.
    B. Venous hum heard over the upper abdomen.
    C. Bruit heard over the liver.
    D. Friction rub.

29. Which of the following would be considered a normal finding when elicited during percussion of the abdomen?

    A. Dullness over the left upper outer quadrant during deep inspiration.
    B. Hyperresonance over the liver.
    C. Tympany over the stomach.
    D. Dullness predominating over the lower quadrants.

Answers to Questions from page 145

13. **(C)** Cholecystokinin and secretin tend to stimulate accessory organs (the gall bladder, pancreas, and liver) while suppressing gastric function. Glucagon acts on liver, muscle, and fat cells to increase blood sugar. Gastrin's primary effect is to stimulate the secretion of HCl.

14. **(B)** Although both cholecystokinin and vasoactive intestinal peptide also augment pancreatic bicarbonate secretion, secretin is the most potent of the three. Cholecystokinin is a neuroendocrine substance, and vasoactive intestinal peptide is probably a neurotransmitter. Secretin is a hormone.

15. **(A)** Insulin decreases the blood sugar by facilitating movement of glucose into cells and by preventing glucose production. In addition, insulin promotes the formation of protein, fat, and glycogen, which also decreases the blood sugar. Secretin and gastrin act primarily on the gastrointestinal tract and have less direct effect on blood sugar levels.

16. **(D)** Glycogen is stored carbohydrate. Glucagon is a hormone produced by the alpha cells of the pancreas. Its role is to increase the blood sugar (glucogenesis) by breaking down glycogen (glycogenolysis), not by forming it (glycogenesis). Another way it increases the blood sugar is through gluconeogenesis (making glucose out of stored fat and protein).

17. **(A)** Branches of the celiac artery supply the stomach, esophagus, and duodenum, which are the sites of upper gastrointestinal bleeds. The superior mesenteric artery supplies the rest of the small intestine and the proximal colon. The inferior mesenteric supplies the distal colon. The portal system is a venous system.

18. **(B)** The efferent vessels (or vessels leading away from) the liver are the hepatic veins. The hepatic arteries supply the liver with oxygenated blood, and the portal veins carry blood from the gastrointestinal tract to the liver; they are both afferent. The hepatic ducts are not vessels; they drain bile formed in the liver toward the gall bladder and duodenum.

30. Palpation of the normal liver is expected to reveal

A. Guarding with deep palpation.
B. A lower border 5 cm below the costal angle.
C. A very soft, compliant inferior edge.
D. An irregular surface.

31. Which of the following laboratory values is/are the most specific for hepatocellular damage?

A. Prothrombin time (PT) and partial thromboplastin (PTT) time.
B. Alkaline phosphatase level.
C. Glutamic oxalate transferase (SGOT) and glutamic pyruvic transferase (SGPT) levels.
D. Amylase level.

32. The least invasive method used to diagnose pancreatic pseudocysts is

A. Ultrasound.
B. Endoscopic retrograde cholangiopancreatography (ERCP).
C. Peritonoscopy.
D. Percutaneous transhepatic cholangiography (PTC).

33. The loss of which gastrointestinal fluid is most likely to lead to metabolic alkalosis

A. Bile or pancreatic fluid.
B. Gastric fluid.
C. Small intestinal fluid.
D. Large intestinal fluid.

34. Which of the following gastrointestinal products contains the highest amount of bicarbonate?

A. Gastric secretions.
B. Small intestinal secretions.
C. Bile.
D. Pancreatic secretions.

Answers to Questions from page 146

19. (D) Parasympathetic nerve fibers innervating the gastrointestinal tract originate primarily from the vagus nerve and are found in both cranial and sacral spinal nerves. They secrete acetylcholine. Both sympathetic and parasympathetic nerves are distributed in the inner and outer walls of the intestine.

20. (D) Acinar cells secrete enzymes for digestion and bicarbonate to buffer the acid contents entering the duodenum from the stomach. They are stimulated by the vagus and by the hormones secretin and cholecystokinin. Insulin and glucagon are secreted by the islets of Langerhans.

21. (A) Fats are emulsified by bile. Lipase is also involved in fat digestion, but its role is to break down triglycerides. Amylase is involved in carbohydrate digestion, and gastrin is a hormone that helps to regulate digestion.

22. (C) Bilirubin is a breakdown product of hemoglobin, and its production is increased in hemolytic anemia. The liver as well as the rest of the reticuloendothelial system can hemolyze red blood cells. The liver can conjugate bilirubin before releasing it into the blood stream, whereas the rest of the system cannot. Urobilinogen is produced by the intestines from conjugated bilirubin, and only a portion is absorbed and excreted by the kidneys.

23. (C) In biliary tract obstruction, the major outlet for conjugated (direct) bilirubin made by the liver is lost, and therefore, the amount released into the blood stream is elevated. The level of unconjugated (indirect) bilirubin goes up whenever hemolysis is increased owing to an increase in bilirubin production by tissues unable to conjugate it. Urobilinogen is decreased in biliary tract obstruction, because the bile does not reach the intestine, where the urobilinogen is made. Both indirect and direct bilirubin is eventually elevated in hepatocellular damage and extrahepatic obstruction, but the percentage of conjugated bilirubin is usually higher in the latter situation.

35. The most direct evidence that the patient is currently in a catabolic state is the fact that

    A. Today's weight is 1 kg less than yesterday's.
    B. The 24-hour urinary creatinine is decreased.
    C. The nitrogen balance is negative.
    D. An anthropometric evaluation is below normal standards.

36. Signs of immnosuppression in malnourished patients include

    A. Leukocytosis.
    B. Increased hypersenstivity to skin tests.
    C. Delayed reactions to skin tests.
    D. Sepsis.

37. One of the possible complications of parenteral nutrition administration is

    A. Hypoglycemia.
    B. Hyperosmolality.
    C. Overhydration.
    D. Edema.

38. Which of the following untoward laboratory findings is most likely to occur during parenteral nutrition administration?

    A. Metabolic alkalosis.
    B. Hyperkalemia.
    C. Hyperphosphatemia.
    D. Hyponatremia.

Answers to Questions from page 147

24. (**D**) Kupffer cells are macrophages of the immunologic defense system. They are a major factor in detoxification of the blood stream and remove quickly most of the bacteria entering the portal system, before it enters the central circulation. Synthesis of clotting factors and metabolism of fat, carbohydrate, and protein are accomplished by the hepatocytes, not the Kupffer cells.

25. (**C**) Inflammatory diseases of the abdomen (cholecystistis, appendicitis, pelvic inflammatory disease) are often well localized. When an abdominal organ is distended (as in intestinal obstruction), the pain is usually difficult to localize and not as sharp but is characteristically cramping (waxing and waning).

26. (**D**) The only normal movements seen on inspection of the abdomen are ventilatory motion, seen especially in men, and epigastric pulsations, seen in thin individuals. Superficial veins and peristalsis are not normally visible.

27. (**B**) Normal bowel sounds occur at the rate of about 5–35 per minute. When intestinal obstruction occurs, they first change to louder, faster, tinkling borborygmi. Later, as the bowel muscle weakens and the disease progresses, bowel sounds are diminished or absent. Peritoneal friction rubs may occur later if peritonitis develops.

28. (**B**) Portal hypertension may cause increased portal vein resistance and a resultant hum. A succussion splash may be heard over a fluid- and air-filled stomach when the patient's abdomen is shaken. A bruit is caused by arterial turbulence, and friction rubs are caused by inflamed peritoneal membranes. Neither is necessarily a consequence of portal hypertension.

29. (**C**) The only finding listed that may be normal is tympany over the stomach, which can occur if the stomach is empty or air-filled. Dullness over the left upper quadrant on inspiration suggests splenomegaly. The liver is normally dull to percussion, and the gastrointestinal tract (lower quadrants) is usually hyperresonant or tympanic.

39. An intervention that may reduce the risk of aspiration from enteral alimentation would be to

    A. Keep the head of the bed flat and the patient turned to the side.
    B. Use intermittent rather than continuous feedings.
    C. Use small-bore feeding tubes.
    D. Increase the infusion rates.

40. The drug of choice for relief of severe pain in patients with pancreatitis is

    A. Morphine sulfate.
    B. Meperidine.
    C. Cholinergic agents..
    D. Salicylates.

41. The statement that correctly characterizes peptic ulceration of the duodenum is

    A. It is less common than that of the stomach.
    B. It is rarely the cause of severe upper gastrointestinal bleeding.
    C. It may be the result of injury to the mucosa from decreased histamine release.
    D. It is sometimes assoociated with hyperplasia or hypersensitivity of the oxyntic cells.

42. The pathophysiology of stress ulcers may be related to

    A. Decrease in blood flow to the gastrointestinal mucosa.
    B. Increase in the mucosal barrier by aspirin or alcohol.
    C. Increase in regeneration of gastric mucosa.
    D. Cholinergic inhibition.

43. The assessment tool(s) that most reliably diagnose(s) the source of an upper gastrointestinal bleed is (are)

    A. The history and physical examination.
    B. Laboratory measurements.
    C. Endoscopic examination.
    D. Barium radiologic studies.

Answers to Questions from page 148

30. (**A**) In order to feel the edge of a normal liver, the hand is placed under the right costal margin and directed upward toward the right shoulder. The examiner pushes down and then toward the diaphragm while the patient inhales, so that diaphragmatic contraction pushes the liver down. In a normal patient, the liver will not be felt without fairly firm pressure, which may elicit pain. It will feel firm, not hard or soft, and fairly smooth.

31. (**C**) SGOT and SGPT, although elevated in other disorders, are the most likely to be elevated in hepatocellular damage. The PT and PTT are important indicators of the patient's risk for bleeding, but they may be elevated in many other disorders and fairly normal in early liver damage. The alkaline phosphatase more directly reflects biliary obstruction, while amylase is used to assess pancreatic function.

32. (**A**) Diagnosis of a well-localized pseudocyst usually requires nothing more than ultrasound or computerized axial tomography (CAT) scanning; the latter is more expensive. ERCP may be used to yield more information in a patient whose symptoms do not subside and in whom surgery is being considered, but it is a more invasive technique. Peritonoscopy with ultrasound is occasionally used to drain the cyst. PTC allows visualization of the route of bile flow from the liver to the duodenum and would not specifically reveal a cyst.

33. (**B**) Gastric fluid is high in hydrogen (acidotic) and in potassium. Loss of either hydrogen or potassium may cause metabolic alkalosis, although it is rarely severe. Small intestinal fluid, bile, and pancreatic fluid are higher in bicarbonate. Bicarbonate loss may lead to metabolic acidosis. The large intestine normally produces very little fluid.

34. (**D**) One of the roles of pancreatic secretions is to buffer the acidic chyme entering the duodenum. It contains very high levels of bicarbonate (approximately 120 mEq/L) and its pH (8.0 or above) is alkaline. Bile and small intestinal fluid are also fairly alkaline but do not contain as much bicarbonate as do secretions from the pancreas.

44. The most important goal in the treatment of bleeding duodenal ulcers is

    A. Stabilizing the patient to prepare for surgery as soon as possible.
    B. Administering intra-arterial vasopressin to effectively decrease all blood flow to the area.
    C. Replacing volume losses to stabilize hemodynamics.
    D. Administering intravenous histamine antagonists to decrease bleeding from the ulcers present.

45. Which of the following is a possible indication for surgical intervention in a patient with bleeding peptic ulcers?

    A. The loss of over ¼ of the patient's volume in 3 days.
    B. The need for massive transfusions in the first 24 hours.
    C. Successful stabilization by medical therapy.
    D. The presence of stress ulcers.

46. The autodigestion that occurs in pancreatitis is thought to be primary caused by

    A. Fat breakdown products.
    B. High-protein exudates.
    C. Activated trypsin.
    D. Calcium precipitates.

47. Possible precipitating factors in pancreatitis include

    A. Certain types of hyperlipidemia.
    B. Hypocalcemia or hypoparathyroidism.
    C. Intrahepatic biliary tract obstruction.
    D. Renal failure.

48. A patient with acute pancreatitis most often presents with which of the following findings?

    A. Pronounced abdominal rigidity.
    B. Nausea and vomiting.
    C. Gray-Turner's or Cullen's sign.
    D. Ascites

Answers to Questions from page 149

35. (**C**) Nitrogen balance measurements are made to assess metabolism. When nitrogen intake is above nitrogen output, the patient is more than meeting metabolic demands and is in positive nitrogen balance, or an anabolic state. When the nitrogen intake is below the nitrogen output, the patient is not meeting metabolic demands and is in negative nitrogen balance, or a catabolic state. Daily weight fluctuations may be reflecting recent fluid volume changes. Urinary creatinine levels decrease with decreased muscle metabolism and also with decreased glomerular filtration rates. Because a single below-normal anthropometric measurement may reflect a chronic problem, it should be repeated serially to evaluate current trends.

36. (**C**) The immune response mediates the normal response to skin test antigens. Immunosuppression may be evidenced by decreased or delayed reactions. The ability to raise the leukocyte count indicates a functioning, not suppressed, immune system. Sepsis is a complication rather than a sign of susceptibility.

37. (**B**) Depending on the glucose concentration, osmolality of parenteral nutrition solutions can be as high as eight times the serum osmolality. Fluid may be shifted by osmosis from the interstitial and cellular spaces to the blood stream and then lost through a glucose diuresis, leading to dehydration. There may be a transient hypervolemia (increased blood volume) but not overhydration (increase in total body fluid volume). Hypoglycemia is less likely to occur from administration of high glucose solutions than from abrupt discontinuation of the solution or from overzealous coverage with insulin.

38. (**D**) Parenteral nutrition can lead to hyperchloremia. Because a rise in chloride forces the bicarbonate down, the end result may be metabolic acidosis. Whenever glucose goes from the blood stream into the cell or into the nephron, potassium and phosphorus may be drawn along with it, causing hypokalemia or hypophosphatemia. Hyperglycemia is often accompanied by dilutional hyponatremia, as fluid is attracted by osmosis into the vascular space. (*Note*: Remember the suffix *emia* refers specifically to states in the plasma.)

49. Laboratory manifestations that would indicate pancreatitis include

    A. An elevated serum amylase level with a low pancreatic isoamylase-to–total amylase ratio.
    B. A low amylase-to–creatinine clearance ratio.
    C. An elevated urinary amylase.
    D. Markedly elevated liver function values.

50. The treatment of a patient with pancreatitis may be expected to include which of the following?

    A. Codeine to control the pain.
    B. Anticholinergic or antienzyme agents to suppress pancreatic function.
    C. Prophylactic antibiotics to prevent abscess formation.
    D. NPO in the acute phase and a low-fat diet in the resolution phase.

51. One of the hallmarks of the general pathology of hepatitis is

    A. Necrosis more pronounced in the hepatocytes than in the Kupffer cells.
    B. Intrahepatic biliary tract obstruction.
    C. Extrahepatic biliary tract obstruction.
    D. Isolated lobar involvement.

52. An immunologic laboratory test that can be used to diagnose the presence of the hepatitis-B virus is

    A. Anti-HAV (IgM).
    B. Anti-HAV (IgG).
    C. HBs Ag.
    D. HAV in the stool.

53. The typical clinical presentation for hepatitis B consists of

    A. Familial exposure with an insidious onset.
    B. Familial exposure with an abrupt onset.
    C. Parenteral exposure with an insidious onset.
    D. Parenteral exposure with an abrupt onset.

Answers to Questions from page 150

39. **(C)** The risk of aspiration is reduced if the solution is administered via smaller, less irritating tubes that will not disturb the competence of the lower esophageal sphincter. Continuous feeding at slow rates is less likely to cause regurgitation than intermittent or high-rate infusion. Although turning the patient to the side is protective, keeping the head flat is not.

40. **(B)** Meperidine and morphine both may relieve the pain, but morphine may cause spasm of the papilla of Vater and decrease the flow of pancreatic secretions. Because cholinergic agents do not decrease pain and may stimulate the pancreas, they are contraindicated. Salicylates are not potent enough for severe pain and may irritate the gastrointestinal tract.

41. **(D)** An increase in the number or sensitivity of oxyntic or parietal cells can cause hypersecretion of gastric acid, beginning a vicious circle that can lead to peptic ulcers. Increased levels of gastric acid stimulate release of histamine, which in turn triggers further gastric acid secretion. Peptic ulcers are much more likely to occur in the duodenum than the stomach and are the most common cause of severe upper gastrointestinal bleeding.

42. **(A)** Theories of mechanisms that lead to gastroduodenal ulceration include ischemia (decreased blood flow), decreased effectiveness of the mucosal barrier (aspirin or alcohol), decreased regeneration of mucosal cells, and increased gastric acid secretion. Vagal or cholinergic stimulation can trigger the latter.

43. **(C)** The history and physical examination may reveal that the patient is bleeding but do not reveal the site. Laboratory measurements help assess the amount of blood loss (hematocrit and hemoglobin) and the severity of shock (arterial blood gases) but also do not reveal the site. If endoscopy can be performed, the bleeding lesion can often be visualized and possibly treated. Barium studies are difficult to do during an acute bleed and, although they may reveal an ulcer crater, cannot readily detect whether or not it is the source of the bleeding.

54. A common finding during the acute phase of viral hepatitis A is

    A. Mild hepatomegaly.
    B. Splenomegaly.
    C. Weight loss.
    D. Serum sickness.

55. What abnormal laboratory finding is most often the first indication that a patient may have viral hepatitis?

    A. Elevated alkaline phosphatase.
    B. Elevated IgM and IgG.
    C. Elevated transaminases.
    D. Elevated indirect bilirubin.

56. The complication most likely to occur with hepatitis A is

    A. Death.
    B. Fulminant hepatitis leading to failure.
    C. Chronic hepatitis.
    D. Post-hepatitis syndrome.

57. One of the measures recommended to protect persons exposed to patients with viral hepatitis is

    A. Strict isolation precautions, especially during the icteric phase.
    B. Blood precautions, especially for hepatitis B.
    C. HBIG for those with anti-HB present in serum.
    D. Hepatitis A vaccine.

58. Hepatic encephalopathy can occur

    A. When ⅔ of the liver tissue has been destroyed.
    B. During stable early phases of Laennec's cirrhosis.
    C. With severe hepatotoxicity.
    D. From low-protein diets in patients with cirrhosis of the liver.

Answers to Questions from page 151

44. (**C**) The main goal of therapy is to replace volume losses while trying to control bleeding. The vast majority of patients stop bleeding spontaneously and do not require surgical intervention. Measures thought to help control bleeding tendencies include intragastric lavage (controversial) and intra-arterial vasopressin administration. The problem with vasopressin in duodenal hemorrhage is that it does not constrict all of the blood supply. Histamine antagonists may improve healing but do not decrease active bleeding.

45. (**B**) Although the criteria are not well standardized and each patient must be considered individually, commonly quoted indications for surgery include transfusion requirements over 1500 ml, loss of over 30% of the estimated blood volume in the first 24 hours, and breakthrough bleeding during appropriate immediate medical care. Stabilized patients rarely require surgery, and stress ulcer is one of the most difficult types to control surgically.

46. (**C**) Autodigestion can occur when trypsin, elastase, or phospholipase is activated. Fat necrosis, high-protein exudates, and calcium binding are consequences, not triggers, of the pathologic process.

47. (**A**) Type I, IV and V hyperlipidemias are associated with an increased risk or pancreatitis. The same is true for hyperparathyroidism. Hypocalcemia, hypoparathyroidism, and renal failure are possible complications of pancreatitis, not causes. In order to obstruct flow from the pancreatic duct, the obstruction must be distal to where the pancreatic duct merges with the common bile duct, i.e., extrahepatic rather than intrahepatic.

48. (**B**) The majority of patients present with severe radiating epigastric pain, nausea, vomiting, and fever. The pain is not usually associated with pronounced abdominal rigidity. Ascites and Gray-Turner's or Cullen's signs may occur but are fairly rare.

59. Manifestations of cirrhosis of the liver include

    A. Hyperaldosteronism and hypergonadism.
    B. Low mixed venous oxygen tension.
    C. Decreased spinal cord reflexes.
    D. Decreased serum colloid osmotic pressure.

60. Which of the following findings becomes apparent during the later stages of hepatic encephalopathy?

    A. Asterixis.
    B. Constructional apraxia.
    C. Dysarthria.
    D. Stupor and severe disorientation.

61. One of the studies done to monitor the degree of liver dysfunction rather than its causes or complications is

    A. Serum transaminase measurement.
    B. Alkaline phosphatase measurement.
    C. Ultrasound.
    D. Electroencephalogram.

62. Interventions used specifically to decrease serum ammonia levels in patients with hepatic encephalopathy include *all but* which one of the following?

    A. Administration of enteral neomycin.
    B. Administration of lactulose.
    C. Restriction of protein intake.
    D. Restriction of hepatotoxic agents.

63. Esophageal varices would be *least* likely to develop in patients with

    A. Celiac artery hypertension.
    B. Portal hypertension.
    C. Portal vein thrombosis.
    D. Cirrhosis of the liver.

Answers to Questions from page 152

49. (**C**) Although laboratory manifestations of pancreatitis are not highly specific or sensitive, an early elevation of serum amylase (2–3 days) and more prolonged elevation of urinary amylase (5–7 days) are suggestive. The pancreatic isoamylase-to–total amylase ratio and the amylase-to–creatinine clearance ratio would both be high, not low. Liver function values will not be markedly elevated unless there is associated hepatic disease.

50. (**D**) In order to reduce stimulus of the pancreas, the patient will usually be NPO for the acute phase and dietary fat will be restricted for several weeks. Codeine is not the agent of choice for pain because of its possible spasmotic effect on the sphincter of Oddi. Anticholinergic and antienzyme agents have not been proven effective, and antibiotics are contraindicated unless an effective organism has been identified.

51. (**A**) The damage that occurs in hepatitis is primarily to the hepatocyte and not to the reticuloendothelial or Kupffer cell network. It is widespread and not confined to a single lobe. Neither intrahepatic nor extrahepatic obstruction is likely.

52. (**C**) HAV in the stool is the first finding seen in hepatitis A. Serum anti-HAV (IgM) and anti-HAV (IgG) elevate later in its course. HBs Ag is a test for hepatitis B. HAV stands for hepatitis A virus. HBs Ag stands for hepatitis B surface antigen.

53. (**C**) Hepatitis A is more likely to be transmitted through oral-anal routes or familial exposure, whereas hepatitis B is more likely to be transmitted parenterally. Hepatitis A has a shorter incubation period and a more abrupt onset than hepatitis B.

64. It has been observed that surgical shunting procedures in the treatment of esophageal varices

    A. Are better used to prevent bleeding from varices than to cure it once it has started.
    B. Are associated with less mortality than medical therapy alone.
    C. Are preferred over sclerotherapy at this time.
    D. May lead to hyperdynamic state.

65. Which method of treatment for bleeding esophageal varices can be performed at the bedside via endoscopy?

    A. Distal splenorenal shunt.
    B. Sclerotherapy.
    C. Transhepatic obliteration of varices.
    D. Esophageal stapling.

66. Cancer of the esophagus

    A. Has a comparatively good prognosis.
    B. Usually occurs in the upper third of the esophagus.
    C. Often metastasizes to the brain.
    D. Is rarely symptomatic until late in the course of the disease.

67. The earliest signs or symptoms of cancer of the esophagus frequently include

    A. Dysarthria.
    B. Substernal fullness when eating.
    C. Shortness of breath on exercise.
    D. Lymphadenopathy.

68. Postoperative care of patients undergoing surgical procedures for esophageal cancer involves

    A. Maintaining a negative nitrogen balance.
    B. Administering drugs to decrease the gastric pH.
    C. Reducing reflux esophagitis by elevating the head of the bed.
    D. Prohibiting the use of any tubes that pass through the esophagus.

Answers to Questions from page 153

54. (**A**) Hepatomegaly, splenomegaly, nausea, vomiting, and abdominal pain are all symptoms of any form of viral hepatitis. Hepatomegaly and splenomegaly may both occur in the acute phase, but mild hepatomegaly is far more common. However, any significant hepatomegaly suggests a problem other than hepatitis, such as cirrhosis or tumor. Weight loss occurs later in the course of hepatitis, and serum sickness is a feature of hepatitis B.

55. (**C**) The transaminases—SPGT (or ALT) and SGOT (or AST)—are markedly elevated in the majority of patients with viral hepatitis. Alkaline phosphatase may be slightly increased. Immunoglobulins are increased in a minority of cases. The bilirubin level often rises, but usually, direct bilirubin is more elevated than indirect bilirubin.

56. (**D**) Post-hepatitis syndrome is the most common complication listed and can occur in any form of hepatitis. Fulminant hepatitis and death are less common and are primarily a consequence of hepatitis B. Chronic hepatitis does not occur after hepatitis A.

57. (**B**) Both parenteral and enteric isolation precautions are taken in patients with suspected hepatitis. However, the patient is less infectious in the icteric phase than in the pre-icteric phase. Blood precautions are more important for hepatitis B than hepatitis A. If an exposed person is positive for anti-HB, immunity is present and HBIG is not indicated. A hepatitis A vaccine has not been developed to date, and protection can be provided only by immune serum globulin given promptly after exposure.

58. (**C**) One setting for hepatic encephalopathy is acute hepatotoxicity. It does not occur in Laennec's cirrhosis until the disease has progressed to the end stage, unless the patient's liver function is challenged by an unstabilized event. Relatively low-protein diets are used to decrease the risk of encephalopathy. Even early symptoms of liver disease do not appear until 3/4 of the tissue is destroyed.

69. Surgical intervention for cancer of the esophagus is the treatment of choice

    A. As soon as the diagnosis is made.
    B. Because it offers the best chance of a cure.
    C. Only when the upper third is involved.
    D. As a palliative measure in a minority of patients.

70. The body's response to peritonitis may involve

    A. Decreased third spacing of fluids.
    B. Alkalemia.
    C. Weight loss.
    D. Oliguria.

71. One possible cause for functional ileus is

    A. Hyperkalemia.
    B. Severe blunt trauma to the abdomen.
    C. Cancer of the colon.
    D. Volvulus.

72. The early clinical presentation of obstruction of the large intestine includes

    A. Vomiting and third space fluid losses.
    B. Marked distention and prolonged pain.
    C. Vomiting and marked distention.
    D. Decreased bowel sounds and hypervolemia.

Answers to Questions from page 154

59. **(D)** The inability of the liver to synthesize albumin leads to low serum colloid osmotic (oncotic) pressure. Reflexes are more likely to be hyperactive than hypoactive. In patients with changes in small vessels, pulmonary vasodilation may cause arterial hypoxemia but not necessarily low venous oxygen tensions because of the accompanying hyperdynamic state. Increased cardiac output leads to decreased oxygen extraction and increased venous levels. Aldosterone and gonadal hormone levels may decrease.

60. **(D)** Asterixis (flapping of the hand when the wrist is hyperextended), constructional apraxia (inability to draw simple figures), and dysarthria (problems with articulation, such as slurred speech) all occur in stages I and II of encephalopathy. Stupor and severe confusion are features of stage III.

61. **(A)** The serum transaminase (SGOT and SGPT) levels are used to assess liver hepatocyte function. Alkaline phosphatase measurement and ultrasound are more helpful in diagnosing obstruction. The electroencephalogram is used to help grade encephalopathy.

62. **(D)** Avoiding hepatotoxic agents is obviously appropriate for these patients but is not a measure that specifically reduces ammonia levels. Neomycin and lactulose decrease the amount of ammonia that can be absorbed from the gastrointestinal tract. Restricting protein intake limits the ammonia produced by protein metabolism.

63. **(A)** Esophageal varices occur when blood is shunted into the veins of the lower esophagus from the portal venous system, which normally brings its flow to the liver. Such shunting can occur in portal vein thrombosis or in portal hypertension, a possible sequela of cirrhosis. The celiac artery brings oxygenated blood to the upper gastrointestinal tract, and its blockade does not produce the venous varices.

73. A patient with carcinoma of the pancreas may present with

    A. Symptoms relatively early in the course of the disease.
    B. Pain typical of pancreatic disorders.
    C. Weight gains due to fluid retention.
    D. A history of a known carcinogenic trigger.

74. A tumor of the pancreas located in the head of the pancreas

    A. Is an unusual finding.
    B. May cause a rise in bilirubin and alkaline phosphatase.
    C. Is associated with dark, tarry stools.
    D. Is a contraindication to surgery.

75. Compared with partial resection, a possible disadvantage of total pancreatectomy is that

    A. It is more complicated.
    B. Its complication rate is higher.
    C. The tumor is usually well-localized within the pancreas, thereby making total resection unnecessary.
    D. The patient will develop pancreatic insufficiency after it is performed.

Answers to Questions from page 155

64. (**D**) The central shunting of blood flow and the decrease of vascular resistance may lead to increased cardiac output. A patient with chronic cirrhosis may already have a hyperdynamic system, and hemodynamic support may be necessary. Surgical shunts pose a significant risk and, because not all patients with varices bleed, are not used prophylactically. They have not been shown to decrease the mortality rate, whereas sclerotherapy may do so. Currently, sclerotherapy is preferred over shunts.

65. (**B**) Sclerotherapy is performed by approaching the varix using a fibroptic endoscope and directly injecting a sclerosing agent. Transhepatic obliteration is percutaneous, not endoscopic. Esophageal stapling is done as part of surgical resections. Distal splenorenal shunt is a surgical decompression of the portal system.

66. (**D**) Because cancer of the esophagus is usually at a fairly advanced stage once it is symptomatic, it is often diagnosed late, and the prognosis is poor. The area most frequently affected is the middle third of the esophagus. The upper third is the least often involved. The lung and the liver are the most common secondary sites of metastatic disease.

67. (**B**) The most common chief presenting complaint is dysphagia, often accompanied by a feeling of substernal fullness. Dysarthria and lymphadenopathy are less commonly seen. Shortness of breath may occur late, depending on the site of the tumor and areas of metastasis.

68. (**C**) Elevating the head of the bed is a simple intervention that can reduce reflux esophagitis, a common problem in patients with cancer of the esophagus who have had their lower esophageal sphincter areas surgically removed. Because of this tendency, drugs may be used to increase the gastric pH. Healing is encouraged by meeting nutritional needs as reflected by a positive nitrogen balance. Nasogastric and other specially designed tubes are used to decompress the area to promote healing.

69. (**D**) Only a minority of patients in the United States with cancer of the esophagus undergo surgical procedures. Surgery is most likely to be helpful as a palliative measure in patients with distal lesions, although it is sometimes used for medial or even proximal tumors. To date, a cure has not been developed for this disease.

70. (**D**) Oliguria may result from hypovolemia and decreased renal blood flow as well as increased ADH. Fluid can shift from the vascular space to the peritoneal cavity, leading to an increase in third space volume without loss of weight. Acidemia may occur from metabolic acidosis related to shock and from respiratory insufficiency when diaphragm excursion is limited.

71. (**B**) A possible manifestation of blunt trauma to the abdomen is functional or paralytic ileus. The term implies that the decreased motility is a matter of physiologic dysfunction, rather than anatomic obstruction as occurs with cancer or volvulus. Hypokalemia decreases motor activity of the gastrointestinal tract and may cause paralytic ileus, whereas hyperkalemia may increase motor activity.

72. (**B**) Marked distention and prolonged pain and constipation are more likely to be present in early obstruction of the large intestine. Vomiting and third space fluid losses are more common in small intestinal obstruction. Decreased bowel sounds can occur in both, but hypervolemia does not.

73. (**B**) One of the first signs of carcinoma of the pancreas may be the pain typical of pancreatitis, which is epigastric and radiates to the back. However, symptoms do not occur until late in the course of the disease, and the prognosis is poor. As in many other types of cancer, weight loss is more likely than gain. A few carcinogenic factors are suspected, but none has as yet been positively linked to this disease.

74. (**B**) The most common site for carcinoma of the pancreas is the head of the pancreas. The tumor may obstruct both the pancreatic and common bile ducts, leading to elevations of bilirubin and alkaline phosphatase as well as incomplete digestion of nutrients. Some of the resultant changes seen in the stool are a lighter color and the presence of fat; the stool does not become dark and tarry. Surgery is indicated in selected patients.

75. (**D**) Although many patients with partial procedures also develop pancreatic insufficiency, total resection insures insufficiency. However, these metabolic changes can be managed, the procedure is less complex, and the complication rate is lower. Another reason total pancreatectomy may be advocated is that pancreatic carcinomas are usually multifocal.

Bibliography

American Association of Critical-Care Nurses: Core Curriculum for Critical Care Nursing, 3rd ed. W. B. Saunders Co., Philadelphia, 1985.
An outline of the basic knowledge base of critical care nursing. Contains information from which these questions are written.

Forlaw, L., Bayer, L. M., and Pack, B. (eds.): Symposia on Nutrition. Nurs. Clin. North Am. *18*, 1983.
A collection of articles describing the nutritional requirements of patients with disorders of various systems. Nursing management is emphasized.

Guyton, A. C.: Textbook of Medical Physiology, 6th ed. W. B. Saunders Co., Philadelphia, 1981.
A frequently cited and long-respected advanced physiology resource. The content supplements the more intermediate content of Core Curriculum for Critical Care Nursing.

Kinney, M. R., Dear, C. B., Paca, D. R., and Voorman, D. M. N.: AACN's Clinical Reference for Critical-Care Nursing. McGraw-Hill Book Co., New York, 1981.
A complete reference for critical care nursing comprising anatomy, physiology, pathophysiology, patient management, and procedures of many disorders, including acute gastrointestinal disorders.

Luckmann, J., and Sorensen, K. C.: Medical-Surgical Nursing, A Psychophysiological Approach, 2nd ed. W. B. Saunders Co., Philadelphia, 1980.
A basic but complete reference for medical-surgical nursing. Common gastrointestinal disorders are covered in the framework of a nursing approach.

Roberts, C. J. C. (ed.): Gastrointestinal Disease. Springer-Verlag, New York, 1983.
Overview of adult abdominal disorders. Content can be understood by the beginning practitioner.

Shoemaker, W. C. (ed.): Critical Care, State of the Art, Volume 5. Society of Critical Care Medicine, Fullerton, Calif., 1984.
A selection of key lectures presented at the Society of Critical Care Medicine's 1984 meeting with discussions of nutrition and substrate utilization in the acutely ill.

Shoemaker, W. C., Thompson, W. L., and Holbrook, P. R.: The Society of Critical Care Medicine: Textbook of Critical Care. W. B. Saunders Co., Philadelphia, 1984.
An excellent review of the current practice of critical care medicine. Each chapter is well-written at an in-depth level by an expert on the topic. Acute gastrointestinal disorders are included.

Sleisenger, M. H., and Fordtran, J. S. (eds.): Gastrointestinal Diseases, 3rd ed. W. B. Saunders Co., Philadelphia, 1983.
An advanced, complete resource on gastrointestinal diseases by physician contributors well-respected in their fields.

Sreenivas, V. I.: Acute Disorders of the Abdomen. Springer-Verlag, New York, 1980.
Concise description of the key concepts in diagnosis and treatment of common acute abdominal disorders. A good quick reference.

8 □ PSYCHOSOCIAL IMPLICATIONS

HELEN C. BAIRD

1. Six weeks ago, Mrs. Jones was informed that she had terminal cancer and has approximately 6 months to live. During her morning bath, she said to the nurse, "I've just bought a Mercedes Benz. Hopefully, God will just let me live long enough to pay it off." Which of these stages of the grief process should be the basis for the nurse to plan care for this patient?

   A. Isolation.
   B. Anger.
   C. Bargaining.
   D. Depression.

2. June Taylor is an 8-year-old child with behavioral problems admitted for possible appendicitis. Her mother is quite anxious and talks angrily to the nurses because she feels that the nurses blame her for June's problems. Which of these would be the best interaction by the primary nurse?

   A. Explain to Mrs. Taylor that her anger is difficult for the staff to handle and that it is causing them to avoid June.
   B. Recommend an institutional placement for June as soon as hospitalization is completed.
   C. Convey acceptance of June and avoid blaming the family for her behavior.
   D. Obtain a social service consult for Mrs. Taylor and spend time with June when she is away.

3. Mr. Seas is a chronically ill alcoholic who has just been transferred from I.C.U. His self-concept is very low, and he has begun to discuss his feelings of hopelessness with the 3–11 nurse on duty. This nurse can best communicate her confidence in Mr. Seas' ability to overcome his difficulties by:

   A. Informing Mr. Seas that people in Alcoholics Anonymous can cure him.
   B. Encouraging Mr. Seas to concentrate on his positive attributes and successes.
   C. Increasing responsibility in Mr. Seas through action-oriented behavior.
   D. Reminding Mr. Seas that his family and the staff are there to help him solve his problems.

4. Mrs. Rich, a very attractive 30-year-old woman, underwent a radical mastectomy of the right breast 5 days ago. She refuses to see her three children or her husband. She cries constantly and appears depressed. In planning care for this patient, the nurse should recognize that Mrs. Rich's reactions may be a result of her:

   A. Anticipating feelings of rejection and being unloved.
   B. Psychic pain related to her desire to have children and nurse a baby.
   C. Viewing her disability in proportion to her functional loss.
   D. Fear of dying of cancer.

5. Mrs. Calloway is a 38-year-old vice president of a large corporation. She has been admitted for evaluation of severe migraine headaches. Nursing intervention regarding the pain associated with migraine headaches will be based on which of these statements?

   A. Cranial vasoconstriction precedes migraine pain.
   B. Vasodilatation has no effect on migraine pain.
   C. An aura is never experienced with migraine pain.
   D. There are no physiologic changes that contribute to migraine pain.

6. Which of the following statements made by Mrs. Calloway (see question 5) during the admission assessment would *not* assist the nurse in planning care for her?

   A. "The headaches started 6 months ago when I was promoted to the position of Vice President."
   B. "My mother has had migraine headaches all her life."
   C. "I met a lady one summer who has to take Vitamin B_2 shots for the rest of her life."
   D. "Raising three teen-aged children keeps my nerves on edge all the time."

7. Treatment for physical or emotional illness may sometimes require hospitalization and may induce feelings of helplessness in a patient. Which of these statements should the nurse emphasize for a patient to help him or her develop a positive view of hospitalization?

   A. Hospitalization often disrupts daily routines, preferences, and, at times, biological rhythms.
   B. Hospitalization can increase anxiety and impede progression toward wellness.
   C. Care delivered by a number of health care workers may strip a patient of his individuality.
   D. The emergency equipment and trained personnel found in hospitals can make it a secure place where basic needs can be met.

8. Mr. Garrett has been hospitalized for the past 3 weeks with a diagnosis of chronic cirrhosis of the liver. When the nurse explained to Mr. Garrett that he was going to be transferred to a med.-surg. unit, he appeared panic-stricken and replied, "What's the use! Why not just leave me here?" Which of these actions by the nurse would best alleviate this apparent crisis for Mr. Garrett?

   A. Tell him that the bed is needed for a seriously ill patient.
   B. Encourage him to discuss his feelings with his doctor.
   C. Assure him that all patients are scared of leaving MICU.
   D. Explore with Mr. Garrett how he handled previous life stresses.

9. Two days after suffering a nearly fatal myocardial infarction, Adam Marshall states, "I'm feeling much better. I plan to go home in the morning." The nurse's response will be based on the recognition that the patient is using which of these defense mechanisms?

   A. Denial.
   B. Rationalization.
   C. Projection.
   D. Sublimation.

Answers to Questions from page 161

1. **(C)** The bargaining state can be viewed by the person as a reward for doing the best one can under the circumstances. Mrs. Jones may extend her life by her planning to pay for the expensive automobile.

2. **(C)** The nurse is the primary care person who has 24-hour contact with the patient and family. Trust, rapport, and, if possible, a positive relationship should be established with family. Parents feel a tremendous amount of guilt about behavioral problems in their children. Answer A or B would further isolate the mother's involvement with the health care team.

3. **(C)** If a person is given tasks he can perform, his sense of confidence will increase, tending to help him deal with difficulties. Because hope and self-esteem are interrelated, an increased sense of accomplishment will increase self-esteem. Patients should always retain a voice in their treatment rather than being given the signal that someone else will do it.

10. Mr. Ashton has chronic back pain that is not relieved by analgesics or physical therapy. When he appears in the emergency room in acute distress, nursing intervention should be based on which of these statements?

A. Acute pain cannot be related to chronic illness.
B. Pain can be defined only by the person who is feeling it.
C. Chronic pain never manifests in acute phases.
D. Intensity of the pain is of minimal significance in treatment.

11. Mr. Daley has rheumatoid arthritis. He says to the nurse angrily, "My doctor wants me to remember all the details about my pain! He thinks I'm stupid. It's like he doesn't believe me!" Which of the following suggestions would it be most helpful for the nurse to make to Mr. Daley?

A. Keep a diary about your pain and what measures relieve it.
B. Call the doctor each time you have pain and relate the details.
C. Relay information to your wife so she can keep the doctor informed.
D. Seek a second opinion since you think your doctor is incompetent.

12. Mrs. Johnson is a 37-year-old mother of four children who had a left mastectomy 6 days ago. Both her husband and her children are very attentive to her needs. She stated to the nurse, "I still have pain in my left breast!" The nurse should assess the remark as

A. Pain from patient's incision line.
B. Phantom limb pain following traumatic surgery.
C. A hallucinatory experience.
D. Acceptance of her surgery.

13. Thirteen year-old Kim Samuel was admitted to ICU after suffering severe trauma in an automobile accident. Her right leg was amputated at the knee. Nursing intervention should *first* be directed toward helping the patient adjust psychologically to which of these changes?

A. Inability to dance.
B. Peer rejection.
C. A prosthesis.
D. Body image.

Answers to Questions from page 162

4. (**A**) In general, the greater the disfigurement, the more somatopsychic influence will be felt. Often feelings of rejection and being unloved are associated with disfiguring surgery in females who value beauty and physical wholeness.

5. (**A**) Cranial vasoconstriction does precede migraine pain. When it ceases, vasodilatation occurs, and blood vessels dilate beyond their normal size, whereupon pain occurs. An aura is experienced with migraines if the retinal artery is involved. The disease process is real and is not just in the mind of the person. Physiologic changes such as those associated with stress and anxiety can precipitate or aggravate psychogenic disease processes.

6. (**C**) The pathophysiology of psychosomatic disorders is related in part to the fact that emotional stress finds expression in vascular structures during periods of stress. A person develops a psychosomatic disorder if emotional conflicts are present and emotional outlets are blocked so that these feelings are internalized. Individuals can learn these patterns, and previous history or illness can influence the development of this disorder, so answers A, B, and D contain significant statements.

14. One of the nurse's basic tasks with adolescents is to help them master this developmental stage. In order to promote self esteem of an adolescent, the nurse should:

   A. Avoid limit-setting actions.
   B. Allow the adolescent to maintain control in all situations.
   C. Avoid maternal, punitive, or judgmental actions.
   D. Provide experiences that will decrease the adolescent's feelings of superiority.

15. According to Erik Erikson's eight stages of development, the developmental task of adolescence is to establish a sense of:

   A. Identity.
   B. Generativity.
   C. Ego integrity.
   D. Trust.

16. Mr. Stone is admitted to a detoxification unit in alcohol withdrawal. Which of the following symptoms should the nurse recognize as typical of alcohol withdrawal?

   A. Fear, disorientation, coarse tremors, sweating, and hallucinations.
   B. Sneezing, yawning, watery eyes, severe abdominal cramps, and fine tremors.
   C. Pallor, agitation, dry warm skin, and headache.
   D. Asterixis, drowsiness, nausea, vomiting, and diarrhea.

17. Which of the following characteristics would the nurse expect to find while obtaining a history on an alcoholic client such as Mr. Stone (see question 16)?

   A. He shows a remarkable lack of concern for other people.
   B. He shows a genuine interest in the nurse and is quite charming.
   C. He talks openly about how his behavior has caused problems and asks for help in changing it.
   D. He talks about close friends he has had since childhood.

Answers to Questions from page 163

7. (**D**) This attitude toward hospitalization would help patients as well as personnel to perceive the experience from a positive perspective. The controlling aspects of hospitalization can be threatening and foster a sense of helplessness in a patient. If the patient understands the purpose of such an environment, he or she will likely be more willing to comply with this temporary situation.

8. (**D**) If there are no relatives or significant others, the nurse can explore previous ways a patient may have handled loss, other life crises, and his philosophy of life in order to help him to cope with this situation. Answers A, B, and C would discount the patient's feelings and would not support him in this stressful situation.

9. (**A**) Denial is the first stage of the grieving process. The use of denial as a defense mechanism protects the ego and says to the patient, "This cannot have happened to me."

18. Mr. Stone's wife complains to the nurse of her husband's recurrent alcoholic binges. She says that they disrupt the family and pleads with the nurse for help. The best nursing intervention for a family in this type of crisis is to:

A. Reinforce reality and maintain control while protecting the patient from himself and others.
B. Answer their questions but avoid getting involved, as these families have a reputation for manipulative behavior.
C. Tell Mrs. Stone that she cannot accept total responsibility for her husband's behavior and that she should force him to do so.
D. Provide physical care and refer to a member of the mental health team to meet the family's other needs.

19. Mrs. Case had a vaginal hysterectomy 4 months ago and is now admitted to the hospital for depression. Which of these statements would be useful for the nurse planning care for this patient?

A. Removal of the uterus causes premature menopause.
B. The average woman experiences dysparunia following a hysterectomy.
C. Husbands believe a hysterectomy increases a woman's libido.
D. As with any surgery, a hysterectomy can aggravate existing health problems.

20. Which of the following statements should the nurse include when giving sexual counseling?

A. Sexual abstinence in youth is advised to prevent guilt feelings later in life.
B. Emissions hasten old age and precipitate illness such as cardiac conditions and high blood pressure.
C. Child-molesting and sexual deviations are more common among older men.
D. It is not unhealthy to become sexually active at an early age, because this tendency can be continued later in life with adult sexual expression.

Answers to Questions from page 164

10. (B) The patient's perception of the pain cannot be verified by someone else. Understanding the severity of pain helps in the decision of how to treat the pain.

11. (A) A record helps patients and those involved in their care to understand more about pain and to better control pain relief. Patients have a tendency to recall events as they want to remember them, not necessarily as they actually occur. Keeping a written record of pain experiences could promote more effective communication between doctor and patient and would foster the patient's self-esteem by encouraging participation in his own care.

12. (B) Experiencing pain in a limb or breast after it has been surgically removed is phantom pain.

13. (D) Body image combined with ego identity, the perception of the physical self, shapes how one feels about oneself as a person; alterations of body image can cause severe psychological trauma. Acceptance of body image changes in an amputee would be an initial priority in nursing intervention. A, B, and C are not critical priorities at this stage, but may later emerge as problems related to altered body image.

21. Mr. Smith is a 28-year-old schizophrenic patient hospitalized for angina pectoris. Because of the excessive auditory stimulation in the I.C.U., there has been a regression in his illness. Which of the following is the *most* appropriate nursing intervention for Mr. Smith?

    A. Criticize his testing-out behaviors such as hostility, negativism, and withdrawal.
    B. Establish a behavior modification program to eliminate his inappropriate behavior.
    C. Attempt to intervene before hallucinations occur, and distract him from his delusions.
    D. Obtain an order to use earplugs to lessen the auditory stimulation.

22. Which of the following therapeutic modalities should the nurse recognize as the best to treat an 18-year-old male recovering from drug overdose and dependency?

    A. Individual therapy sessions to increase insight into behavior.
    B. Family therapy to make members aware of client's problem.
    C. Group retreat with individuals of all ages and a variety of problems.
    D. Peer group of ex-addicts to provide strong role identification.

23. Keith is a 19-year-old who has had a long-standing problem with conduct. In the hospital he often pits staff against staff and staff against family. Which of the following nursing goals is most appropriate for Keith?

    A. He will have a consistent and firm limit-setting environment.
    B. He will have a nurse who assumes a mother-surrogate role.
    C. He will receive a high level of empathy from the staff when he cries and makes threats.
    D. He will be allowed close contact with other patients who can meet his needs.

Answers to Questions from page 165

14. (**C**) When dealing with adolescents, nurses should set limits, maintain control of the situation, and avoid being manipulated. They should provide constructive experiences in interactions and should not reinforce negative feelings such as inferiority. Being maternal and punitive can block establishment of rapport.

15. (**A**) A sense of identity is developed during the adolescent period. Generativity is developed between the ages of 25 and 45 years, in young adults. A sense of ego integrity is developed between 50 years and death, in middle and old age. The most important task in infancy is development of a sense of trust.

16. (**A**) Other options describe a patient experiencing withdrawal from drugs, such as heroin, cocaine, and methadone.

17. (**A**) Although the antisocial personality characteristic of an alcoholic is quite charming, the alcoholic lacks the ability to be genuinely interested or concerned. He fails to learn from past experiences and develops superficial relationships with significant others.

24. The doctor has recommended therapy for Mr. Nelson's family during his hospitalization for diabetes mellitus. There appears to be a high level of stress within the family. At the first therapy session Kevin, aged 14, shouts "It's all Melissa's fault. She's making Daddy sick!" The other family members agree with Kevin. Which of these statements should be the basis for nursing intervention with this family?

    A. It is common for family dynamics to assign a scapegoat role within the family system.
    B. Scapegoats are uncommon within family therapy sessions.
    C. This is typical brother-sister rivalry.
    D. The statement should be ignored.

25. The nurse providing therapy for the Nelson family notes that the family reacts as if it were a unit. Like individuals, families attempt to maintain a steady state. In utilizing this concept in assessment, the nurse would expect to observe

    A. Family members attempting to maintain balance by using their previously established behavior patterns during the crisis.
    B. Family disintegration secondary to Mr. Nelson's hospitalization.
    C. New communication patterns among family members.
    D. Family members maintaining equilibrium only through their covert actions.

Answers to Questions from page 166

18. (**A**) In crisis intervention, mobilization of one's strengths and ability to control the situation are needed. Answer B would be inappropriate at any time. Answer C is one of the basic problems underlying alcoholism: the alcoholic does not accept responsibility for his behavior. Physical care is rarely needed except in acute phases or with those individuals suffering brain damage from alcohol abuse. Answer A is the best possible action under these circumstances.

19. (**D**) Answers A, B, and C are myths regarding hysterectomies. Some husbands believe a woman's sexuality decreases rather than increases after hysterectomy. Some women falsely believe they are sexually destroyed by a hysterectomy. Only answer D is a correct scientific interpretation.

20. (**D**) Answers A, B, and C are commonly held myths regarding sexuality. In his sexual research, Kinsey found the content of answer D to be true.

26. Julie Carson, 13 years old, is admitted to I.C.U. for evaluation of cardiac status secondary to severe chest pains at home. The doctor suspects psychosomatic illness. Julie's mother appears unduly anxious and refuses to leave her bedside. The I.C.U. nurse learns from Mr. Carson that his wife has always doted on Julie and made Mr. Carson feel useless in these situations. Which of the following interventions could help the Carson family cope with this crisis?

   A. Mobilize Mr. and Mrs. Carson's mutual support in caring for Julie.
   B. Explain to Mrs. Carson that Julie is tired of her excessive attention and is using her illness to teach her a lesson.
   C. Inform Mr. Carson that Julie wants more attention from him and that she will improve if he gives it to her.
   D. Encourage Mr. Carson to ignore the situation for now.

27. Johnny Carr is an 8-year-old admitted to the hospital for a fractured right leg. He is described by friends and family as a "holy terror" and labeled "disturbed." Which of the following interventions constitute an appropriate short-term goal for nursing management of Johnny?

   A. Assist the Carr family to be a more functional unit.
   B. Have the nursing staff assume responsibility for Johnny's behavior.
   C. Increase Johnny's involvement with the extended family.
   D. Make Johnny a better-behaved child.

28. Three days ago, Mr. Kephart, a 40-year-old white male, was admitted to the hospital for the first time. He complained of sharp, stabbing, precordial chest pain and has requested morphine for relief four times since admission. The nurse notices that Mr. Kephart experiences pain immediately after his wife leaves him alone. Nursing intervention for Mr. Kephart's pain would be influenced by the nurse's ability to recognize that this type of pain is consistent with

   A. Dressler's syndrome.
   B. Malingering.
   C. Psychogenic pain disorder.
   D. High level AV block.

Answers to Questions from page 167

21. (C) I.C.U. environments tend to isolate an individual from normal activities that promote reality orientation. Hallucinations usually begin in an anxious lonely person. The content of hallucination replaces having no "helping" person around. Delusions are false beliefs that cannot be changed by reason. Focusing the patient's attention and stressing reality are the best interventions to prevent environmentally induced hallucinations.

22. (D) Answers A and B would not be advisable for recovering addicts, because such modalities could cause problems with authority figures in individual and family therapy. Answer C would not be beneficial, because an addict gives little credit to behaviors of those who have not had similar life experiences.

23. (A) Answers B and D would be inappropriate in dealing with this patient because they would foster client dependency needs and allow him to manipulate others for his own gain. Answer C would encourage further manipulation and increase staff turmoil as staff became exhausted by his manipulative behavior. Answer A would assist in providing a therapeutic milieu.

29. Mr. Swaggert is a 36-year-old Viet Nam veteran. He is seen in the emergency room for evaluation of a broken right arm. During his admission assessment, he remarks to the nurse, "Even though the war is over, they still control my mind." The nurse will recognize that the patient is experiencing a(n)

    A. Delusion.
    B. Hallucination.
    C. Somatization.
    D. Illusion.

30. Mrs. Smith is a 74-year-old grandmother who is diagnosed as having liver cancer. Her main support system appears to be her three grandchildren, who are very attentive and caring. She expresses to the nurse her feelings of loneliness and futility. To help Mrs. Smith renew her sense of meaning in life and decrease her feelings of loneliness, which of the following nursing interventions would be appropriate?

    A. Encourage Mrs. Smith to knit her grandchildren sweaters.
    B. Tell Mrs. Smith that loneliness is an integral part of old age.
    C. Allow Mrs. Smith to work out her own solutions.
    D. Have Mrs. Smith write down her thoughts for her grandchildren.

31. Mrs. Peters is seen in the emergency room. She is crying uncontrollably at first but then tells you that she has just received word that her mother has died. Nursing intervention will be based on recognition that Mrs. Peters is experiencing which of the following crises?

    A. Developmental.
    B. Situational.
    C. Phenomenological.
    D. Deterministic.

Answers to Questions from page 168

24. **(A)** During crises, family members often single out an "identified person" to be the scapegoat or the cause of problems; in this case, Melissa is the family scapegoat. Because of the involvement of other family members, sibling rivalry would not be the likely mechanism in this situation.

25. **(A)** The family unit acts to achieve balance in relationships even when it is threatened. Family communication patterns help to reveal the degree of balance maintained within the unit. Answer A describes the only situation in which balance can be maintained through verbal and nonverbal behavior.

32. Which of the following should be the nurse's goal for intervention with Mrs. Peters (see question 31) during her crisis?

    A. Help Mrs. Peters to gain insight into her behavior and to admit her mother is dead.
    B. Restructure Mrs. Peters' personality to help her cope with this stress.
    C. Assist Mrs. Peters with problem-solving and maintaining her functioning within her family and community.
    D. Help Mrs. Peters understand that she is having a crisis.

33. Which of the following actions would be most appropriate for the nurse to take in crisis intervention with Mrs. Peters (see question 31)?

    A. Obtaining extensive factual data regarding the incident and Mrs. Peters' usual method of coping with stress.
    B. Convincing the patient that help is available and that treatment starts where she is at the moment.
    C. Explaining to Mrs. Peters that crises have no time limits, so that danger of mental decompensation will be present for a long time.
    D. Encouraging the patient not to make decisions until the crisis is resolved.

34. Mr. Hobbs, a 75-year-old male, is admitted to C.C.U. for 2nd-degree heart block (type II) and is being evaluated for implantation of a permanent pacemaker. The nurse notices that Mr. Hobbs has no visitors. When the physicians make rounds, they talk about the patient, but ignore his presence and make no physical or verbal contact. Which of the following goals represents a means to minimize Mr. Hobbs' sensory deprivation?

    A. Make Mr. Hobbs an active participant in his treatment regimen.
    B. Prevent Mr. Hobbs from getting upset, which could cause him to go into complete heart block.
    C. Divert Mr. Hobbs' attention from the seriousness of his condition.
    D. Determine Mr. Hobbs' knowledge about his disease and condition.

Answers to Questions from page 169

26. **(A)** Murray Bowen observed that in families in which parents were emotionally close, more invested in each other than either was in the child-patient, the patient improved. When parents are close, they are usually consistent in their management approaches, and this consistency increases a child's feeling of security. This situational crisis can be managed most effectively if both parents participate by supporting each other as well as their child.

27. **(A)** According to family therapists, a dysfunctional marital relationship is the main contributor to a disturbed child. It is thought that a disturbed child needs his symptoms to hold the family unit together. It is the nuclear family, not grandparents or other extended-family members, who contribute most significantly to a child's behavior.

28. **(C)** The malingering patient is under voluntary control of his symptoms and has a specific goal in mind. Pain is not a feature of high level AV block, and the pain described is not characteristic of Dressler's syndrome. Psychogenic pain is pain inconsistent with anatomic distribution of the nervous system, is under involuntary control, and has a temporal relationship to environmental stimuli. Mr. Kephart's feelings of loneliness after his wife leaves seem to precipitate his pain.

35. Mr. Carr, a patient recovering from an acute myocardial infarction, remarks to the I.C.U. nurse, "None of you think I'm going to live!" The nurse's response is based on recognizing that Mr. Carr is utilizing which of these defense mechanisms?

   A. Repression.
   B. Projection.
   C. Illusion.
   D. Regression.

36. After receiving tracheostomy care, Mr. Gary requests in a whining manner that he be shaven. Which of these defense mechanisms is Mr. Gary probably using?

   A. Regression.
   B. Denial.
   C. Rationalization.
   D. Projection.

37. Mr. Kelly is a retired colonel who vigorously resists following even routine hospital procedures. He is admitted to the hospital with abdominal pains. Proctoscopy is scheduled for the next morning. A nursing intervention planned at decreasing the patient's feelings of powerlessness in relation to the necessary tests would be to

   A. Assign an orderly to administer the necessary prep.
   B. Allow Mr. Kelly the option of refusing the prep.
   C. Teach Mr. Kelly how to administer his own prep.
   D. Ask Mrs. Kelly if a family member could assist him with the prep.

38. Mr. Richard was admitted to I.C.U. following a tragic automobile accident in which his wife was killed. When questioned about the accident, Mr. Richard replies, "I don't want to talk about this right now. It is too upsetting!" Nursing intervention with Mr. Richard should be based on the nurse's recognition that the patient is using which of these defense mechanisms?

   A. Repression.
   B. Regression.
   C. Depersonalization.
   D. Suppression.

Answers to Questions from page 170

29. (A) *Delusions* are false beliefs that can not be changed by reason; they frequently involve mind control and reference to nonspecific pronouns such as "he" or "they." *Hallucinations* are sensory perceptions that occur without external stimulation. An *illusion* is a misconception of a real external stimulus; no external stimulus precipitated Mr. Swaggert's response. *Somatization* is exhibition of physical symptoms as a result of repressed anger.

30. (D) Nurses cannot find meaning in life for their patients but can mobilize patients' support systems and encourage them to explore meanings for themselves. Answer D could help restore meaning to Mrs. Smith's life by engendering a deepening relationship between her and her grandchildren. Answer A would only temporarily placate Mrs. Smith and would not resolve her feelings in regard to the situation. Answer B is incorrect, as loneliness can affect any age group, not just the elderly.

31. (A) There are two types of crisis. Developmental crises are common to all and involve such events as marriages, death, and divorce. Situational crises occur around random events such as illnesses and accidents. Answers C and D are not types of crisis.

39. The I.C.U. nurse performs a mental status evaluation on a patient with COPD. He remarks, "Don't waste your time. It's no use anyway! I'm not going to suffer like this any longer!" Which of these nursing actions would be most appropriate at this time?

    A. Obtain an order for Elavil for the patient.
    B. Allow the patient more control in his care.
    C. Encourage the patient to set goals for the coming year.
    D. Explore the patient's response for suicidal tendencies.

40. Mr. Reaves is admitted to the C.C.U. for evaluation of chest pains. His behavior is inappropriate, and he uses words that apparently have meaning only for him. Mr. Reaves says, "It's only my eloquacia!" The nurse's initial response to this remark should be to

    A. Ignore the statement and continue with the conversation.
    B. Distract him by changing the topic of conversation.
    C. Consult with his wife for interpretation of his remark.
    D. Ask Mr. Reaves what he means by the word, as it is unfamiliar to you.

41. Mr. Sterns was admitted to the C.C.U. three days ago for evaluation of dizzy spells and brief blackout periods, possibly secondary to pacemaker malfunction. The nurse notices that the patient never mentions his illness, diagnosis, or medications, or the procedures he undergoes. Which of these approaches by the nurse would most encourage the patient to discuss these areas?

    A. "You're always so quiet. Why don't you ever ask about your illness?"
    B. "You are so calm. You don't seem concerned about anything."
    C. "You've got a very good doctor. Why haven't you talked to him about your illness?"
    D. "Patients often have questions or concerns about being sick. If you'd like to talk with us, we'd be glad to answer your questions."

Answers to Questions from page 171

32. **(C)** Crisis theory assumes that the individual in crisis can be "turned around" and that neither he nor the therapist has time just then for insights into causes, psychotherapy into restructuring personality, nor understanding the dynamics of the crisis. The primary goal is to restore the patient's functioning through reestablishing her problem-solving ability.

33. **(B)** Crisis information should be limited to pertinent details. Crises have limits in time and there is a danger of mental decompensation if intervention is not expedited. One of the actions the nurse can take is to help the patient look at options, choose one, and act on it to restore her problem-solving ability.

34. **(A)** Sensory deprivation in the elderly can be induced by situations similar to the one described. Answer B is incorrect; stress does not cause or worsen heart block. Studies have shown that the elderly want to be informed of their treatment and condition, but giving information (answer D) will not diminish sensory deprivation. They are not children but adults, who need to be treated as adults. Diverting their attention (answer C) will not be therapeutic. Making Mr. Hobbs an active participant in his care helps to orient him and involve him with his environment.

42. Mr. Cross was admitted to I.C.U. for acute liver disease. It was noted in his history that he served in the Viet Nam War and was a prisoner of war. On the 11–7 shift, Nurse Rich hears a scream. Going to Mr. Cross' bedside, she observes the patient crying, perspiring, and mumbling over his nightmare about uniformed guards. In handling this crisis, the most appropriate action by the nurse would be to:

   A. Call the hospital security guards to handle Mr. Cross' irrational behavior.
   B. Call the physician and recommend transfer to a psychiatric unit.
   C. Clarify the perceived threat with Mr. Cross and dispel his misperceptions.
   D. Wake Mr. Cross immediately and re-orient him to time and place.

43. Mr. Thompson asks the nurse about some of the beeps and alarms he's hearing in the C.C.U. nurses' station. Which of the following responses would be the best for the nurse to make?

   A. Invite Mr. Thompson to the nurses' station to demonstrate how the alarms are set for upper and lower heart rate limits.
   B. Tell Mr. Thompson to ignore the beeps as they don't affect him.
   C. Close his door so Mr. Thompson is less bothered by the noise.
   D. Cut off all the alarms so as not to disturb the patients.

44. Seventy-year-old Mr. Emery is admitted to I.C.U. to rule out an MI. During his fourth day of hospitalization, the nurse notices that Mr. Emery often turns on his left side when she asks him to turn on his right. The nurse has also noticed his inability to decide what to eat when filling out his menu. Although he seems to be experiencing difficulty processing information, his physical status has remained stable. The nurse should plan nursing intervention for which of these?

   A. Early sensory deprivation.
   B. Pulmonary embolus.
   C. Pneumothorax.
   D. Aphasia.

Answers to Questions from page 172

35. **(B)** Illusion is not a defense mechanism. *Regression* involves returning to an earlier state of development, and *repression* is an unconscious block of memory from one's conscience. In *projection,* a person attributes his own thoughts or feelings to someone else. In this case, Mr. Carr is really the one who thinks he's going to die.

36. **(A)** All answers are defense mechanisms used to cope with anxiety, but denial, rationalization, and projection do not involve the process of returning to an earlier level of emotional development. Mr. Gary displays this behavior of dependency, because he is regressing in his frustrated, anxious state.

37. **(C)** Answers A and D ignore Mr. Kelly's need for independence in his own care and would not decrease feelings of powerlessness. Answer B would not be an option, because failure to prepare the area would render the test results invalid. Answer C would allow this patient some independence in the situation and decrease perceptions of powerlessness.

38. **(D)** *Suppression* is a conscious and deliberate putting out of one's mind thoughts that can be anxiety-producing. *Repression* is an unconscious mechanism. *Depersonalization* is a sense of being someone else. *Regression* is engaging in behavior characteristic of an earlier stage of development.

45. Which of the following nursing actions could diminish Mr. Emery's (see question 44) ability to participate in his own care to the fullest potential?

   A. Offering reassurance and empathy when the patient hasn't asked for it.
   B. Changing the subject when he asks questions that make the nurse feel uncomfortable.
   C. Sharing control of care with the patient and his family.
   D. Removing equipment from a patient after appropriate weaning and support.

46. As a result of hospitalization, Mr. Emery (see questions 44 and 45) is experiencing general adaptation syndrome (GAS), as described by Hans Selye. When assessing this patient for clinical manifestations of physiologic responses to stress, the nurse should recognize that this syndrome is:

   A. An autonomic nervous system and endocrine gland mechanism to help the body fight off stressors and regain equilibrium.
   B. A central nervous system and exocrine gland mechanism that restores homeostasis.
   C. The parasympathetic response to endocrine gland stimulation that helps the body fight stress and restore homeostasis.
   D. The physiologic response of decreasing cardiac output to restore equilibrium.

47. Mr. Tracey, a 43-year-old white male, is hospitalized for his third myocardial infarction. He appears quite depressed and asks, "Am I going to die?" Which of the following is the best initial response by the nurse?

   A. "Think positive thoughts. When patients think they are going to die, they often do."
   B. "It's too early for us to give you an answer to that question."
   C. "That's a question I don't know the answer to, but what do you think?"
   D. "Ask your doctor. He can answer that question better than anyone else."

Answers to Questions from page 173

39. (**D**) The patient has apparently given up hope about his chronic illness and may be making a conscious decision to take his life. Remarks of this nature are classic statements about suicide and require immediate attention. Answers A and B would be inappropriate as priority nursing interventions at this time. The priority is a short-term not long-term goal, so Answer C would be incorrect.

40. (**D**) The ability to trust one's caregiver is a basic need to all patients. Never fool a patient by saying you understand something when you do not. Convey your willingness to understand by being honest.

41. (**D**) Using "why" questions often challenges a patient and blocks further communication about his needs. Answer D approaches the situation from a positive perspective and leads to further discussion.

Questions 48–50 will be based on the following situation:

John Brown is a 14-year-old adolescent admitted to I.C.U. after drinking liquid bleach in a suicide attempt.

48. In an interview with the nurse, John's mother remarks, "He was always threatening to kill himself if he didn't get what he wanted." The nurse knows that

   A. Suicidal individuals rarely give clues to their intentions.
   B. Even casual remarks may be a plea for help that can be followed by the actual suicide.
   C. People who talk about suicide rarely commit suicide.
   D. Anyone who commits suicide is mentally ill.

49. Mrs. Brown (see question 48) remarks, "I guess I've been a lousy parent. I never seem to do anything right!" The nurse's best response would be:

   A. "All parent feel the way you do!"
   B. "Adolescents are impossible. They all act like 2-year-olds."
   C. "There is nothing you could have done. It would have occurred without warning anyway!"
   D. "Raising adolescents is a difficult task even under the best of circumstances!"

50. Dr. Nick informs Mrs. Brown that John actually did not drink an extemely large amount of bleach. Which of the following statements regarding suicidal gestures is *true*?

   A. Suicidal gestures in adolescents are rarely triggered by trivial incidents.
   B. Suicidal gestures can be used in an attempt to influence others or manipulate situations.
   C. If unheeded, suicidal gestures are rarely followed by repeated attempts.
   D. Suicidal gestures are always related to parental conflicts.

Answers to Questions from page 174

42. **(C)** In handling crises produced by fear, the nurse should utilize interaction to clarify perceived threats and reinforce appropriate perceptions of reality. Waking a patient abruptly could cause further regression. Answers A and B would be inappropriate actions for managing a crisis.

43. **(A)** In some instances, demonstrating the functioning of equipment can help the patient tolerate the equipment rather than be anxious about it. Answer C would discredit his anxiety and offer no explanation of his question. Answer B would discount his original question and would be a harsh and uncaring response by the nurse. Answer D would be a negligent and unsafe nursing action.

44. **(A)** The symptoms listed are indicative of sensory alterations seen in sensory deprivation. If the patient were experiencing pulmonary embolus or pneumothorax, there would be definite acute signs and symptoms. There are no indications of a speech disorder.

Questions 51–55 will be based on the following situation:

Mr. Carey, 60 years old, was admitted to I.C.U. for a head injury. The physician has ordered the patient turned only to his right side and back to protect the area from pressure. After the first week, Mr. Carey begins to show signs of mental confusion, even though his physical condition has improved. The doctor and nurse concur that Mr. Carey is suffering from alterations in his sensory level.

51. When assessing Mr. Carey for sensory deprivation, the nurse should

   A. Determine the sensory level to which the patient is accustomed.
   B. Know that patients cope better with continuous periods of sensory stimulation.
   C. Recognize that one's optimum level of sensory input remains constant.
   D. Increase the amount of sensory input without regard to high-input periods.

52. Which of the following statements regarding sensory overload and deprivation is *true*?

   A. Sensory deprivation is solely responsible for hallucinations in individuals with sensory disturbances.
   B. Lack of clarity in thought and illusions occurs only with sensory overload.
   C. Sensory overload can produce symptoms similar to those of sensory deprivation.
   D. Illusions and hallucinations rarely occur in sensory disturbances.

53. Because of Mr. Carey's injury, he is forced to assume a recumbent position. The nurse knows that a recumbent position:

   A. Is the optimum position for decreasing sensory deprivation.
   B. Distorts visual images and auditory perceptions, thereby aggravating sensory alterations.
   C. Has no effect on the patient's spatial environment unless he is wearing eye patches.
   D. Can cause pressure sores but has no effect on sensory levels.

---

45. (**B**) If you do not answer a patient's question, the patient will tend to think one of two things: either that the nurse is incompetent and does not know the answer or that his condition is more severe than it really is. The other options are appropriate nursing actions to maximize the patient's potential.

46. (**A**) The sympathetic, not central, nervous system is responsible for GAS, which consists of a fight/flight response; the release of epinephrine causes a feedback response in the endocrine system to maintain and restore the body's equilibrium. Answer C is incorrect, because it is a sympathetic, not parasympathetic, response. Answer D is incorrect because cardiac output is not decreased in the stress response.

47. (**C**) A nurse must be willing to listen to what the patient says, regardless of the discomfort the nurse is experiencing. If a patient gives verbal or nonverbal clues that the subject of dying is on his mind, the nurse should give him the opportunity to talk about death.

54. Prior to the onset of sensory deprivation, patients often complain of:

    A. Illusions.
    B. Hallucinations.
    C. Delusions.
    D. Boredom.

55. An appropriate nursing intervention in response to Mr. Carey's sensory disturbance would be to:

    A. Move Mr. Carey's bed so he can see the nurses' station more easily.
    B. Play music Mr. Carey enjoys, to stimulate his senses.
    C. Spend brief periods of time sitting beside Mr. Carey.
    D. Position Mr. Carey so he can hear noise in the hallways and the nurses' station to increase his sensory input.

56. Mr. Dalloway has undergone femoral popliteal bypass surgery. His postoperative course was complicated by respiratory failure and congestive heart failure. Four days of constant physical assessments have resulted in sensory overload. The most appropriate nursing intervention to alleviate this disturbance would be for the nurse to

    A. Schedule the drawing of blood samples to coincide with nursing care, and then allow for quiet periods.
    B. Schedule care so one person would be with the client constantly.
    C. Play soft, continuous music while performing care.
    D. Use touch sparingly as a therapeutic input to diminish sensory overload.

57. Nurse Keith is supervisor of the coronary care unit. Over the past 3 months, she has worked a great deal of overtime. She has become increasingly irritable and complains of feeling fatigued. Staff recognizes that these manifestations could be the result of

    A. Sensory overload.
    B. Cognitive disturbances.
    C. Dementia.
    D. Severe sensory deprivation.

Answers to Questions from page 176

48. (**B**) A common characteristic of suicidal behavior is described in answer B. Answers A, C, and D are myths about suicide.

49. (**D**) Being a parent of a normal adolescent is difficult, but the problems of parents whose children have attempted suicide are much more complex. Parents may have a strong sense of failure; a nurse should show compassion and understanding in these situations. Answer A reflects a lack of understanding of the problem. Answers B and C are not therapeutic responses but reflect a more subjective viewpoint.

50. (**B**) Answers A and C are untrue. Suicidal gestures can be related to quarrels with siblings or peers, and to school problems, as well as to parental conflicts (answer D). Even superficial gestures that go unheeded (answer C) can result in more dramatic attempts at self-destruction.

58. Which of the following interventions would best alleviate Nurse Keith's (see question 57) symptoms?

    A. Playing tennis.
    B. Quiet periods of reading at home.
    C. Jogging with a friend.
    D. Playing bridge.

Questions 59–63 will be based on the following situation:

Mr. Richardson, a 58-year-old engineer, is admitted to the coronary care unit. His wife has accompanied him to the hospital.

59. When Mr. Richardson's wife arrives in the C.C.U., she states angrily to the nurse, "He constantly pushes himself, even though Dr. Kaplan has advised him to slow down!" The nurse's best response would be

    A. "Some individuals have a difficult time changing their lifestyles when they have always been high achievers."
    B. "People never listen to their doctors."
    C. "People sometimes resist change even to the point of pushing themselves to the brink of death."
    D. "Some people never face reality."

60. On the morning following Mr. Richardson's admission, his physician discusses with him the seriousness of the heart damage that he has suffered. After the physician leaves, Mr. Richardson remarks to the nurse, "That doctor is wrong. I'm as sturdy as a bull and plan to return to work next Monday." In order to best respond to Mr. Richardson, the nurse must recognize that which of the following mechanisms is the most likely reason for his remark?

    A. Conscious or unconscious denial of his condition to allay his anxiety.
    B. Lack of knowledge about his heart disorder.
    C. The need for a second medical opinion to eradicate any doubt he may have.
    D. A realistic attitude in view of his not having any pain.

Answers to Questions from page 177

51. **(A)** One's optimum level of sensory input is changeable and dependent upon several factors, including the amount of sensory stimulation one is accustomed to at home and/or work. Individuals tend to cope better if high-input periods are followed by lower levels of input. A busy, aggressive executive would develop sensory deprivation more rapidly than a nursing home resident.

52. **(C)** A thorough assessment is needed in patients with sensory disturbances to determine whether the symptoms are from sensory deprivation or overload. Answer A is incorrect because hallucinations may occur in sensory overload or may stem from pre-existing psychiatric problems. Lack of clarity in thought and illusions (answer B) may occur in sensory deprivation as well as sensory overload. Answer D is incorrect because these disturbances frequently occur in sensory alterations.

53. **(B)** After less than 3 hours of lying in the recumbent position, patients can begin to exhibit signs of sensory deprivation. Answers A, B, and C are factually incorrect.

61. Male patients often associate the heart with masculinity. They view an insult to the heart, such as a myocardial infarction, as an attack on their ability to function. Which of these actions would assist the nurse in determining Mr. Richardson's perception of his illness?

   A. Ask Mrs. Richardson what her husband thinks about his illness.
   B. Assess what immediate fears, feelings, or threats the patient may have as result of his illness.
   C. Review his medical history to determine which past experiences would contribute to his perception of his illness.
   D. Focus on his nonverbal communication, as he cannot verbally express his true feelings.

62. One week following his myocardial infarction, Mr. Richardson complains of mild muscular pain. A review of his chart indicates that for the past 48 hours he has complained of the lights and noise, of feeling tense and tired, and of not being able to sleep. Nursing assessment reveals no changes in his respiratory or circulatory status and no changes in his ECG. Which of these nursing actions would be best?

   A. Administer morphine sulfate gr. 15 I.V. stat.
   B. Initiate independent nursing measures to promote relaxation.
   C. Explain to the patient that anxiety is causing his pain.
   D. Tell him that the pain is nothing to worry about, since his vital signs and ECG have not changed.

Answers to Questions from page 178

54. (**D**) In the early stages of sensory deprivation, patients often complain of boredom. The other responses relate to symptoms occurring after the onset of sensory overload or sensory deprivation.

55. (**B**) Studies show that input provided to relieve sensory disturbances must be meaningful to the patient. Playing music would be an activity meaningful to Mr. Carey. Answers A, C, and D would provide alterations in sensory level, but these changes would not necessarily produce meaningful stimuli for the patient.

56. (**A**) Plan several procedures to be done together, in order to allow the patient periods of low input between periods of care. Individuals cope better if high-input periods are followed by lower levels of input.

57. (**A**) Nurses who work in particularly busy and stressful areas of the hospital such as ER and intensive care areas often feel the effects of sensory overload and exhibit symptoms of fatigue and irritability.

63. While giving discharge instruction to Mr. and Mrs. Richardson, the nurse includes information on when they can expect to resume sexual relations. Mr. Richardson replies, "That won't be a problem, as we gave sex up when I was 42." Which of the following physiologic events may be responsible for declining sexual activity?

A. A decrease in androgen levels normally begins about the age of 40.
B. Males go through a climateric period similar to that in females that results in decreased sexual drive.
C. A decreased estrogen level after the age of 40 decreases the male's sex drive.
D. A decrease in sex drive at about age 40 is a compensatory mechanism that slows down the aging process.

64. Nurses in critical care areas are often confronted with patients who have attempted or considered suicide. Many myths surround this concept. Which of the following statements regarding suicide is *true*?

A. People who talk about committing suicide never do it.
B. Don't let that patient talk about suicide, as it can only put ideas in his head!
C. All suicidal behavior should be seriously considered as it may be a plea for help.
D. Only someone schizophrenic would commit suicide.

Questions 65–67 will be based on the following situation:

Terry is a 23-year-old male who is admitted to the ER following a one-car accident. His lower jaw is broken and his right zygomatic bone has been crushed by the column of the steering wheel.

65. Terry's mother is extremely upset and unable to be of any assistance in providing information. In this situation, the nurse should:

A. Tell other family members they will need to help Terry's mother cope better.
B. Talk to her privately for a few minutes and check on her periodically.
C. Send her home and tell the family to leave a number where they can be reached.
D. Insist that the information is critical and that she must cooperate.

Answers to Questions from page 179

58. **(B)** The symptoms of sensory overload can best be alleviated by quiet periods of reading or quiet walks alone to decrease the level of sensory input. The other options all maintain fairly high levels of sensory stimulation.

59. **(A)** Often, people desperately attempt to hide limitations in an effort to protect their self-concepts. Answer C could cause an unwarranted fear. Answers B and D appear quite trivial and nontherapeutic.

60. **(A)** Commonly, cardiac patients exhibit early denial of the seriousness of their illness. *Denial* is the conscious or unconscious repudiation of all or a portion of the total available meaning of an illness in order to allay anxiety and minimize emotional stress. Answers B and D are inappropriate, because the doctor has discussed the seriousness of his illness. Answer C is inappropriate because the patient appears to be protecting his own ego rather than doubting the medical competency of the M.D.

66. When Terry is discharged from the hospital his jaws are still wired. He has been instructed about his diet of soft and liquid foods. He is given an appointment to return to the doctor's office in 2 weeks for evaluation and plans for plastic surgery to repair his cheek bone. During this period, he refuses to go out of the house and will only allow his mother to assist in his care. Terry's behavior most likely reflects:

   A. Suicidal ideation.
   B. Impaired self-image.
   C. Acute psychosis.
   D. Paranoia.

67. During Terry's appointment with the doctor, plans were made for facial reconstruction that may take as long as 2 years to complete. When working with Terry, the nurse knows that:

   A. Discussing with him and his family the details of the impending stressful operation may help to minimize some family problems before they occur.
   B. It is best to allow the family and significant others to work out their problems as a family unit on their own.
   C. It is best to have the physician explain all of the anticipated needs and problems.
   D. It would be best to suggest that Terry and his family consult a family psychiatrist to assist in the therapy.

68. Mr. Kay has been in I.C.U. for 5 days. Every morning the nurse notices Mr. Kay wringing his hands for 3 minutes. Which of these actions should the nurse take first?

   A. Ask the patient the meaning of his behavior.
   B. Consult with the physician about a means of changing the behavior.
   C. Continue observing for the behavior at other times of the day.
   D. Obtain an order for a sedative to administer when the patient is anxious.

Answers to Questions from page 180

61. **(B)** The patient's perception of his illness includes the knowledge, understanding, fantasies, and misconceptions about it. Listen for the patient's ideas about what caused his illness, because some perceive illness as punishment for past deeds. Both verbal and nonverbal communication modes are important in perception assessment. Answer D assumes that the patient is unable to express his feelings, when in fact he may be capable of doing this. Answers A and C are incorrect, because the perceptions are likely to be biased since they were not obtained from the individual himself.

62. **(B)** After a week of hospitalization, the patient's agitation and insomnia may be related to stimuli in his environment.

69. One goal of intervention when caring for a dying patient is to respond to identified needs of the individual. This goal would be best accomplished by

    A. Guiding the conversation toward the acceptance phase of the illness.
    B. Listening carefully for cues in the conversation to identify the present stage of grieving.
    C. Reassuring the individual that everything possible is being done to ensure his recovery.
    D. Confronting the patient immediately in order to resolve the grief process.

70. Mr. Mason is a 63-year-old mechanic with a long history of alcohol abuse. He had a subtotal gastrectomy about a year ago. He has returned to the hospital with a diagnosis of cancer of the pancreas. He is scheduled for a pancreatoduodenectomy (Whipple) procedure. One evening, Mr. Mason asks, "There won't be much left of me when they finish, will there?" The nurse's best response would be

    A. "Are you afraid to die?"
    B. "That's right Mr. Mason, but you will do fine."
    C. "What do you think your operation will do to you?"
    D. "Not much left of what . . . ?"

71. Following Mr. Mason's operation (see question 70), he does not regain consciousness and the doctor gives little hope of his recovering and returning to his family. In assessing family interactions, the nurse should identify

    A. Previous strengths and supports utilized during family crisis periods.
    B. Which family members are most capable of assisting with Mr. Mason's care.
    C. Appropriate funeral arrangements and close family members to contact.
    D. Any dissatisfactions of nursing care provided for Mr. Mason.

| **Answers to Questions from page 181** |

63. (**A**) Factors responsible for declining male sexual activity include a decrease in androgen beginning in the mid-40's and gradually leveling off at age 60. It is disputed whether males actually experience a climateric, but it is definitely wrong that the sex drive stops. Answer C is incorrect, since male hormones decrease rather than estrogen. Premature cessation of sexual functioning accelerates the physiologic and psychological processes of aging.

64. (**C**) A, B, and D are all myths surrounding suicide and are common remarks made by nonprofessionals. C is the correct answer, as all suicidal behaviors should be considered serious and warrent professional intervention.

65. (**B**) By spending some time with her, the nurse will be able to allay some of the mother's anxiety and provide reassurance. Answer A is incorrect, as this situation requires professional nursing intervention that should not be passed on to family members. Answer C is not a nursing decision. Answer D is inappropriate as it ignores the mother's needs during this crisis period.

72. Which of the following is an important evaluative indicator for effective nursing care of the dying patient?

 A. To document each stage of the dying process accurately.
 B. To assess the acceptance level achieved by patient and family.
 C. To ascertain how the family will cope with problems following the death.
 D. To determine whether the dying process was positively influenced.

73. Paul is the 8-year-old brother of Johnny, who died recently of leukemia. Paul is admitted to the hospital for a tonsillectomy. He asks the nurse, "When I go to sleep, will I go to heaven like Johnny?" The nurse's best response is

 A. "The doctor knows what he's doing. He'll be with you!"
 B. "Tell me more about what happened to Johnny."
 C. "Don't be afraid—you're just having your tonsils out!"
 D. "Have you ever had surgery before?"

66. **(B)** Adolescents are more acutely aware of body image than people of other ages. Regression is evidenced by this behavior, although not to the extent of any psychotic symptom or suicidal tendencies.

67. **(A)** Anticipatory guidelines help families cope with events by discussing the details of an impending stressful occurrence. Answers B, C, and D shunt professional nursing responsibility to the family or physician.

68. **(A)** Before the nurse intervenes, it is necessary to validate behavioral meanings with the patient. According to Peplau, the only relevant basis on which the nurse can formulate a plan of care is to evaluate the meaning of the behavior to the patient. Intervention by any of the other options would be based on assumption.

74. Sibling response to death can range from overt depression to preoccupation about one's own death. Nursing interventions to increase coping ability of siblings would be best accomplished by

    A. Encouraging the sibling to recall only the good and happy times.
    B. Arranging for siblings to be routinely scheduled to care for the dying child.
    C. Providing opportunities for siblings to discuss the illness and death throughout the process.
    D. Allowing the sibling to spend as much time away from home as possible to cope with grieving process.

75. Critical care environments can pose high levels of personal and professional stress in nurses. Which of the following actions would best result in decreasing stress among staff members?

    A. Engaging in constant daily introspection of self with peers.
    B. Establishing relationships within the unit that promote open communication and resolution of conflicts.
    C. Maintaining a detached attitude to reduce the risk of personal involvement with peers.
    D. Establishing relationships with family members of patients to mobilize the nurses' support systems during times of stress.

Answers to Questions from page 183

69. **(B)** The initial assessment in any dying patient is to determine the stage of grieving. From that point, interventions can be established. To confront the patient or offer false reassurance could obstruct appropriate assessment.

70. **(C)** Answer C will determine how much he knows and how much his doctor has told him. The nurse can then proceed to teach or support as needed. Answer A is incorrect, as the nurse is alluding to a conclusion that the patient has not mentioned. Answer B stifles further communication. Answer D is an inappropriate use of reflection, because Mr. Mason has already stated "not much left of me" and this answer could reinforce fears of the situation without appropriate resolution.

71. **(A)** When assessing the needs of the dying patient, it is important to achieve an understanding of the strengths of the family members to cope during previous crisis periods. This will identify and mobilize their current support systems. Answers B, C, and D address only isolated problems and do not take care of the family unit's needs.

| **Answers to Questions from page 184** | **Answers to Questions from page 185** |

72. **(D)** Some individuals never complete all stages of the grieving process; the effectiveness of nursing care cannot be based on whether all stages are completed. The most important intervention is to allow the patient to die with dignity and respect. Any positive influence in the death process can be viewed as effective and appropriate nursing care.

73. **(B)** Answer B is the only response that will provide the nurse with further information by which to determine how much Paul understands about his brother's death. Further interventions and responses would need to be based on this information. Answer D does not address the original question but only diverts the child's attention.

74. **(C)** Answer C would allow increased self-awareness regarding the process of death and help the sibling develop a more positive attitude toward his own mortality. Answer B would be inappropriate, as children may not be capable of giving the care needed. Answers A and D would encourage avoidance of true feelings and would not result in appropriate resolution.

75. **(B)** Mobilizing support systems within the critical care environment can increase camaraderie and assist in coping with a variety of stressful situations common to these areas. Self-awareness and peer evaluation are important but can be destructive if carried to extremes. Answer C isolates the individual and decreases feelings of universality, which are important to critical care areas. Answer D is inappropriate; staff do not seek support from family members.

Bibliography

American Cancer Society: Pain Control: A Guide for People with Cancer and Their Families. American Cancer Society, New York, 1982.
A manual that discusses all aspects of pain and therapeutic approach to pain control and answers practical questions posed by individuals and their families.

American Psychiatric Association: Diagnostic and Statistical Manual of Mental Disorders III. U. S. Library of Congress, Washington, D.C., 1980.
A comprehensive text of the classification of mental disorders. It discusses symptomatology of disorders as well as prognostic significance of the different classifications.

Carter, Frances: Psychosocial Nursing Theory and Practice in Hospitals, Community Mental Health. Macmillan Publishing Co., New York, 1981.
An excellent psychiatric nursing text written from a strong psychoanalytical perspective. Stresses nursing interventions and teaching implications in psychosocial aspects of care.

Clunn, P., and Payne, D.: Psychiatric Mental-Health Nursing. Medical Examination Publishing Company, Garden City, 1981.
A psychiatric nursing text that is well organized and easy to understand for the beginning psychiatric student. Presents material on psychodynamics of the underlying problems and nursing interventions in a straightforward way.

Ellis, J., and Nowlis, E.: Nursing: A Human Needs Approach. Houghton Mifflin Co., Boston, 1981.
Presents nursing theory in depth and detail. The nursing process is introduced, and concepts such as stress and crises are related to the health-illness continuum.

Estes, N. J., and Heinemann, M. E.: Alcoholism: Development, Consequences and Interventions, 2nd ed. C. V. Mosby Co., St. Louis, 1982.
A paperback text strong in research statistics related to current theories of alcoholism. Treats alcoholism as a disease and is written from a preventative health viewpoint. Both authors are nurses.

Everly, G., and Rosenfield, R.: The Nature and Treatment of the Stress Response. Plenum Press, New York, 1981.
Explores the psychophysiologic responses to stress. Describes different theories and treatment modalities appropriate for stress. Strength lies in presentations of Selye's theory of stress and biofeedback modalities.

Giovanni, L.: Drugs and Nursing Implementation. Meredith Corp., New York, 1971.
Paperback that stresses drug interactions and appropriate nursing interventions. Also discusses appropriate teaching implementations related to drug therapy.

Kenner, C., Guzzetta, C., and Dossey, B.: Critical Care Nursing—Body, Mind, Spirit. Little, Brown & Co., Boston, 1982.
An excellent textbook integrating the holistic aspects of critical care with the assessment and management of individuals in this environment. Information is straightforward and concepts are well-defined.

Machlowitz, M.: Workaholics. Addison-Wesley Publishing Co., Reading, Ma., 1980.
Strong in theoretical and practical applications of the stress concept. Provides stress scales, guides, and other indexes for practical application to evaluate stress responses.

Murray, R., and Huelskoelter, M.: Psychiatric Mental Health Nursing: Giving Emotional Care. Prentice-Hall, Englewood Cliffs, 1983.
An excellent psychiatric textbook that correlates current Diagnostic Statistical Manual III terminology. Presents numerous tables and condenses information regarding psychotrophic drugs and psychopathology in easily understood language with a strong emphasis on nursing's teaching interventions. Written from a holistic perspective with enough use of medical science to make the information usable.

Sater, V.: Conjoint Family Therapy. Science and Behavior Books, Palo Alto, 1976.
A paperback that discusses family dynamics from a communications theory approach. Written from a social model, and omits any references to medical science modalities. Straightforward in interventions and can be a useful guide to any professional working with families.